The Medical Day Planner

The Guide to Help Navigate the Medical Maze

TORY ZELLICK

Victory Belt Publishing Inc
Las Vegas

First Published in 2012 by Victory Belt Publishing Inc

ISBN 13: 978-1-936608-77-5

Printed in Hong Kong

Introduction

On March 15, 2009, I found myself sitting on a pristine beach on a small island in the Gulf of Thailand. The scenery was stunning, the water was crystal clear, and the food was lovely, and I was, to say the least, completely miserable. You see, fifty-one days prior to this moment I watched my mother take her final breath.

After a six-and–a-half-year fight, my mother lost her battle with breast cancer. The disease itself had eaten away at her tiny body; leaving her riddled with surgical scars and broken bones as well as cognitively impaired. What the disease was unable to do was crush her spirit, soul, and dignity. She was fifty years young.

At the ripe old age of eighteen, I remember walking into our family living room, just as I had done every day before. My mom was sitting in the same corner of the couch where she always sat with the same book she had been reading the day before, but the vibe in the room was off. She was holding her book as if reading, but in fact, she was only staring at the pages. She looked up at me, smiled, and asked me to take a seat next to her. My heart sank. . . .

"I went to the doctor today," she began. "You know I had found a lump in my breast, right?"

"Yeah," I whimpered with a questioning tone.

"The results of the biopsy confirm that I have cancer."

BAM! I had just received a sucker punch to the gut.

"I will start radiation and chemotherapy this week. Everything will be fine," I remember her promising me as I began to cry like a four year old feeling abandoned on the first day of pre-school. I laid my head in her lap and cried for quite some time. She massaged my scalp like she had when I was much younger. It would be the last time she was the care-giver in our relationship.

The next six and a half years were filled with doctor appointments, surgical procedures, tests, scans, and treatments. I had become the "taxi" mom had always joked about being. She was so pleased on my sixteenth birthday, when I was finally able to drive myself to all of my obligations and she was able to park the family "taxi." The family taxi had downsized from a 1994 Suburban to a 2004 Camry, but the duties still remained.

As the primary caregiver, I was responsible for getting my mom to and from her multiple appointments, as well as being the official "form-filler-outer." We made the best of every day; she continued to be positive and instilled hope in our family. Her strength and the incredible journey we made together as a family unit shaped who my brother, father, and I have become, which leads me back to March 15, 2009.

As I lay on the beach and watched the sunset, I grew more and more lonesome. I was one day shy of my twenty-fifth birthday, and as far as I was concerned, my entire world had come crashing down. I reflected on all of the previous situations I had experienced, questioned the decisions I had made, and began to come to grips with the fact that I would have to learn what my life would be without her. In that very moment, I asked myself "how could my situation have been improved from the beginning?"

The answer was simple: if only our primary physician had handed me a fill-in-the-blank guide to track Mom's care, I could have done a better job. I had done my best to be organized, but the truth is I had no idea what was important to track at the beginning of this journey. The trail was long and full of pot-holes, and I was a novice hiker.

I spent the rest of that night outlining what you are now holding in your hands. The intention of this book is to help instill confidence in your caregiving ability. You may find yourself caring for one of our country's disabled veterans, your twenty-year-old son who was in a terrible car accident, a cousin suffering from a mental illness, your sister who suffered a stroke at the age of fifty, a parent who is starting to show signs of dementia at age eighty-one, or yourself if you have been diagnosed with a condition you are able to manage on your own. You will need an organizational guide. This diagnosis-neutral tool will provide a guide to improve your journey and, most of all, help you keep a positive outlook and a hopeful mind-set.

It is the same determination and positive attitude that my mom shared with me that I hope to share with you. The caregiving road may be difficult, but it can certainly be improved with organization and teamwork.

This book was born out of turning loss into love.

I wish you the best of luck on your journey.

Patient Information

Name..

Address...

Email...

Phone (Home)........................(Work).....................(Cell)..............................

Birth Date...................................Blood Type...

Emergency Contact #1

Name...

Phone (H).........................(W)........................(C)..................................

Relationship...

Emergency Contact #2

Name...

Phone (H).........................(W)........................(C)..................................

Relationship...

Known Allergies..
....

Dietary Restrictions..
....

Diagnosis...
....

Caregiver #1

Name...

Phone (H).........................(W)........................(C)..................................

Caregiver #2

Name...

Phone (H).........................(W)........................(C)..................................

Caregiver #3

Name...

Phone (H).........................(W)........................(C)..................................

Caregiver #4
Name..
Phone (H)...........................(W).........................(C)...............

Caregiver#5
Name..
Phone (H)...........................(W).........................(C)...............

Attorney Name...
Phone...
- ☐ Trust
- ☐ Living Will
- ☐ DNR (Do Not Resuscitate)
- ☐ DNI (Do Not Intubate)
- ☐ Durable Power of Attorney (DPOA)

Name DPOA...
Phone (H)...........................(W).........................(C)...............
Relationship..

Insurance Broker Name...
Phone...
Insurance Company...
Policy #..

Accountant Name...
Phone...

Notary Name...
Phone...

Other Contact...
Phone...

Other Contact...
Phone...

Patient Information

First and foremost, it is important to have all personal information about the patient in this book. The first few lines are very simple: the full legal name of the patient; any previous names the individual may have gone by (marriages, divorces, and adoptions may influence surnames and may help with locating previous medical records); the permanent address of the patient or the address where you would like medical bills sent; and the patient's e-mail address, phone numbers, birth date, and blood type. If you are unsure of the patient's blood type, there are several ways to go about finding this information. If the patient has ever donated blood, the facility in which the blood was donated should have a record of the patient's blood type. The second option is to ask the lab where recent blood tests have been drawn; they should be able to accommodate your request for blood type.

Next are two spaces for emergency contacts. The individuals you choose as your emergency contacts should have access to a phone on a regular basis and be readily available should an emergency occur. The emergency contacts may not necessarily need to be your Durable Power of Attorney (DPOA), as the DPOA information will also be in this section. In some instances the DPOA is not always present for day-to-day activities and is only in a position of decision making from a distance.

Next you will find several lines to document the patient's known allergies and dietary restrictions. Allergies could range from reactions to adhesives on tapes, over-the-counter medications, and prescription medications to the cottonwood tree outside your bedroom window. Write every known allergy the patient has experienced in the past. You may find as you continue down this road of hospitals, medications and treatments that new allergies arise. Continue to document these new allergic reactions in this section of the planner.

Dietary restrictions can be just as important to some individuals as allergies. Many individuals choose not to eat certain foods based on religious, environmental, or social beliefs. Others have an intolerance to foods such as dairy and gluten. Make sure this information is displayed appropriately in this book and communicated to hospital (or facility) staff in the future. Notes can be made in your medical chart so these food substances are avoided during meal time. Depending on the patient's diagnosis—for example, stroke or traumatic brain injury (TBI)—swallowing disorders may occur. Symptoms such as coughing during or after taking a bite of food as well as the inability to clear food from the oral cavity may require the assistance of a Speech-Language Pathologist (SLP). A Modified Barium Swallow (MBS) study will likely be ordered to identify the cause, and dietary restrictions may be recommended. Write these recommendations in this section.

The final lines in the Patient Information section are available for you to write out a detailed description of the patient's diagnosis. Depending on the disease, disorder, ailment, or accident, you may need to note to what "stage" the disease has progressed to, the body location of the problem, and if the problem has metastasized to any other region of the body. Ask the doctor to help you in acquiring the appropriate information about the patient's diagnosis.

Helpful Tip #1: Once you have the correct "lingo" surrounding the patient's diagnosis, you are free to do your own research on the Internet. Please remember that new studies are constantly being done, new information arises every day, and statistics change by the moment. Do not take what you read online for gospel; use it as a guide to find new, insightful questions to ask your physicians and providers.

Caregivers' Name & Numbers

Every situation is different. You may be the only caregiver for this individual. You may be one of seven siblings caring for this individual. Either way, it is important to have a current list of all individuals who are pertinent to making this caring process successful. Have a list of the first and last names of each individual, and each of their phone numbers—work, home and cell. You never know when you will need to get in touch with one of them.

Helpful Tip #2: Once you have the names of all the caregivers written down, make as many photocopies as necessary and distribute the list to each of the caregivers. This book will stay with the patient at all times. If the phone list is copied, every caregiver will have the up-to-date information of the other caregivers.

Attorneys

When people hear the word attorney, it generally brings up negative connotations. People sometimes have personal experiences regarding how they were wronged by an attorney, or they know a friend, or a friend of a friend, who paid an attorney and didn't get the outcome they had hoped for. Everyone has their story.

However, guidance is very important to make sure the legal affairs of an ailing individual are in order, and the preconceived negative notions about attorneys should be set aside. While many issues in this section are difficult to discuss and very easy to put off, certain ones must be addressed while the ailing individual is capable and competent, such as legal decisions and explanations of what he or she envisions with end-of-life choices. Delaying this discussion can result in the involvement of the court, a much more expensive and intrusive experience.

It is also important to remember that, as with all professionals (doctors, accountants, insurance agents, etc.), there are good attorneys and not-so-good attorneys. Finding a personal "fit" with an attorney is essential. You want to feel comfortable talking about all aspects of estate planning, including end-of-life decisions. The appropriate attorney should have extensive experience in estate planning, which generally encompasses wills, trusts, DPOA (durable power of attorney), long-term care planning, and Advanced Health Care Directives.

Do not hesitate to interview (and yes, that is exactly what you should do!) several attorneys to find one you like. Have a list of questions, and make sure that the attorney is able to articulate what each document does, the legal implications of each document, and can actually talk with you on a personal level in language you understand. Ask your friends for referrals.

There are all sorts of legal websites that provide guidance on "do-it-yourself" wills, trusts, "living" wills, and other legal documents. However, they generally provide "boilerplate" forms that only take into consideration the broad overview and do not address issues that are specific to an individual. When you find yourself in the middle of a health crisis, "test driving" generic guides to legal documents may not be appropriate.

This section is simply a brief overview of what documents should be considered and prepared so that the ailing individual can rest easy, knowing his or her desires regarding medical treatment, end-of-life decisions, and distribution of personal and real property at the time of death will be honored. This can be accomplished by having documents that address these matters prepared by an attorney in advance.

Once each document has been prepared, check its box in the personal section of this book.

Advanced Health Care Directive

My close friend's father was a physician. He died approximately five years ago after a prolonged illness. To this day my friend has kept a copy of her father's Advanced Health Care Directive, which is a very well-written document specifically defining what her father thought was "acceptable" health care in the event of a prolonged illness. The first paragraph written by her father starts with: "As a physician who has practiced medicine for over three decades, I write this directive regarding my health care knowing that I fear far more *living when I should have died*, than *dying when I should have lived*." This was followed by very specific instructions about treatment as his illness progressed.

One of the most important decisions an ailing individual can make when contemplating end-of-life decisions is what type of treatments he or she wants or does not want. In this age of amazing medical advances, illnesses that once brought a rapid end are no longer fatal or can be managed over a much longer term. The "natural" end of life can be postponed for several years with medical intervention. Individuals can be maintained on life support with ventilator and feeding tubes for significant periods of time, but some will prefer that those extreme measures not be undertaken. That is why an Advanced Health Care Directive is so important.

An Advanced Health Care Directive is a document that allows an individual to notify his or her physician, family, and friends of personal desires with respect to medical treatment, special treatments, testing, surgery, therapy, and other medical treatment options when that individual is no longer able to make such decisions. It allows the individual to control end-of-life decisions without family members trying to guess the individual's wishes or imposing their own desires for treatment.

It can also include directives stating "do not resuscitate" (DNR) or "do not intubate" (DNI), indicate whether the individual wants his or her organs donated after death, and give instructions about nutrition and hydration when the individual is unable to eat or drink. In addition, it allows an individual to select an agent (spouse, family member, friend, or other individual) to handle the health care decisions in accord with what the ailing individual has set forth in the directive. In a nutshell, it is essentially a document that allows an ailing individual to control personal health care decisions even when he or she is no longer able to speak and/or to deny or consent to treatments.

Individuals who have been diagnosed with a terminal illness need to be able to speak freely with their physicians, family, and friends, and let them know what is important to them when they are dying. For example, does the person wish to remain at home and receive hospice, or would he or she rather be in a skilled nursing home or a hospital? For some individuals, the thought of dying causes great fear and they may wish for all possible treatments. Others may wish to die peacefully at home or in hospice, only receiving palliative care.

It is likely to be helpful for the ailing individual to speak with his or her physician about what the options are for health care treatment at the end of life. My attorney cautions that we should not be too broad with statements of our wishes. His primary example was the unqualified statement "I do not want life-sustaining treatment." Written in this way, this statement could inhibit the use of IV nutrition or hydration, antibiotics, or a temporary ventilator, where such treatments might result in regaining a normal quality of life for years to come. Thus, an Advanced Health Care Directive needs to be specific about treatment options. If the person is unsure of what is best, he or she can speak with family, friends, spiritual counsel, hospice professionals, and others who might be able to provide some thoughts. The ultimate decision is up to the individual. Once the decisions and preferences have been established, they should be shared with the person's physician, family, friends, and designated and alternative agents.

Who Should Act as Your Agent?

This is a personal decision that should be left up to the ailing individual. However, it is important to talk with the proposed "agent" to ensure he or she is willing and able to follow the patient's desires and preferences. For many individuals, it is a family member. For my friend's father, who didn't want the burden of following his directive placed on his children (which would mean making decisions to allow their father to pass away), he chose a very close friend who was also a physician. My friend's father spent hours discussing what he wanted with the agent. To ensure there would be no surprises, he asked the appointed agent to review a copy of the directive with his adult children, who had been provided copies in advance. By making someone who was not a family member the agent, his children were spared making decisions that would be very difficult and emotional.

It is best that a successor agent be named in the event that the initial designee is unable or unwilling to serve when the time comes. Naming multiple co-agents to work together is not recommended, since in the absence of specific instructions, co-agents must agree to all aspects.

What to Do after the Decisions and Preferences Have Been Established

When the ailing person has decided what he or she wants, it is best for the individual to meet with an attorney and have the document drafted to ensure that it is legally binding and correctly sets forth the individual's desires. Laws in each state are different, so it is important that the Advanced Health Care Directive complies with the requirements of the state in which the ailing individual resides.

What should you do with the Advanced Health Care Directive after it has been signed? First and foremost, keep a copy of the completed and signed directive in a place that is safe and easily accessed.

Then, provide a copy of the directive to the following:

1. Your family and your agent (the individual and alternative individuals who are designated to make the decisions for the ailing individual);

2. Your physician;

3. Your health care providers and others who may be there or be called in case of emergency;

4. The hospital or health care institution that provides treatment for the ailing individual.

DNR

DNR is the abbreviation for "do not resuscitate." A DNR document is a binding legal document that states that if an ailing person goes into cardiac (heart) or pulmonary (lung) arrest, resuscitation should not be attempted. This can be included in an Advanced Health Care Directive, as set forth above. However, it should be noted that a DNR does not prevent administration of medication or other treatment. The agent may also make this election at the time of entry to the hospital or facility if the patient is incapacitated.

Again, this is where an attorney is very helpful and legal expertise is required. Different states have different requirements for a DNR to be enforceable. It is not possible to set forth each individual state's requirements here. It is strongly suggested that you contact an attorney to ensure that the documents are valid and legally enforceable.

DNI

DNI is the abbreviation for "do not intubate." If an individual goes into pulmonary arrest, has a significant head injury, falls into a coma, or any number of other events that prevent an individual from breathing on their own, a DNI states that the individual may not be intubated, meaning, usually, placed on a ventilator that "breathes" for the individual. This can also be included in an Advanced Health Care Directive.

What Is Durable Power of Attorney (DPOA) for Financial Affairs?

A durable power of attorney is a document through which an individual can appoint a person, persons, or an organization (agent or "attorney of fact") to manage financial affairs when the individual is unable or unavailable to manage his or her own affairs. This document must be signed by the individual when the individual has the mental capacity (is competent) to understand the nature of the document and its legal implications, and it should be notarized. Again, requirements differ from state to state, so it is imperative that you utilize an attorney. DPOAs are generally prepared when there is a possibility that an individual may become mentally incapacitated due to a specific illness, in which case the individual can specify when the power of attorney goes into effect.

A general power of attorney can be broad and allow your agent to do many things, including managing real property (vs. personal property), investments, and bank accounts; entering into contracts on your behalf; and many other things. Additional powers can be granted through the written document. A power of attorney can also be more specific, appointing an agent to only act in specific situations (for example, you are traveling out of the country and a transaction will be closing in your absence). Needless to say, given the responsibility and authority you are giving to your agent, it is imperative that the agent you choose be honest and someone you trust to make decisions that are in your best interest.

People often get confused about the term "durable" in durable power of attorney. "Durable" here simply means that the document will remain in effect or take effect when the individual becomes mentally incompetent.

The most important thing one needs to remember is that a power of attorney is only valid and legally enforceable if the person signing the power of attorney is mentally competent at the time of signing. The person must have a clear understanding of the power they are granting to another individual and the legal implications. In the event there is any doubt of the competence of the person signing the document, have the person's physician examine him or her and write a letter stating that the individual is competent to enter into the agreement.

Finally, it is imperative that there be a "trigger" for the power of attorney to go into effect. For example, the language in the document can state that it will go into effect when the individual is no longer mentally competent. The definition of "competence" can be set forth in the document, and the individual can determine what is required for him or her to be deemed incompetent. For example, the individual can decide that his or her primary treating physician will determine incompetence or ask that more than one physician make that evaluation. It is likely that the physicians will test the individual to determine whether he or she is able to understand the nature of the transactions and make reasonable decisions about them.

Trusts vs. Wills

There are numerous misunderstandings about the differences between wills and trusts. Both are considered estate planning documents.

Wills are used to distribute property to beneficiaries, specify last wishes, and name guardians of minor children upon death. However, a will is subject to probate proceedings and requires court supervision for handling payments to creditors, beneficiary challenges, and other issues that may arise. There are probate fees, and the matter must be completed in probate court.

Living trusts, also known as revocable trusts, go into effect only after a person dies. However, they are set up during the lifetime of the settlor (person who owns the trust assets). During the settlor's own lifetime he or she acts as the trustee and can make changes to the trust. Essentially, the individual's assets are transferred to the trust, and the assets are then held "in-trust." Any other assets that are not transferred to the trust during the settlor's lifetime can be transferred to the trust upon the settlor's death through a pour-over will. This pour-over will should also be prepared at the time the trust is drafted.

It is imperative that you have an estate planning attorney prepare your will, your trust, and your pour-over will. There are legal requirements, ramifications, and tax consequences of each, and an attorney will provide you with the information and advice necessary to make the best decision and ensure the required formalities are included. This is not the time to be overly concerned about the cost of the document preparation. A good attorney can provide you invaluable information that may save your heirs and beneficiaries significant sums in estate and inheritance taxes.

What Happens If You Do Not Have a Will or a Trust?

If you die without a will or a trust, it means you have died "intestate." There are several ramifications. If you die "intestate," the court decides how your assets are to be distributed pursuant to state law, which generally sets out "intestate succession" for inheritance of your estate assets. Unfortunately, you may not wish to leave anything to the person who would get it according to law. A will prevents that from occurring.

Also think about designating a guardian for your minor children. If you do not designate someone as the guardian and there is not another parent, the state will make that determination as well.

If you die intestate, the court has the authority to appoint an individual to "administer" the estate, as well as provide fees for that administrator, before your estate is distributed.

This information is not meant to scare individuals into hiring an attorney to prepare these documents. However, when you have an established relationship with a good attorney he or she can be very helpful in difficult times. Legal issues vary tremendously from state to state, so it is imperative you receive accurate information and the proper documents to ensure your wishes, desires, and preferences are honored as you reach the end of life.

Medical Insurance Broker

You may or may not have an insurance broker. If you do, this individual may become your best friend. If you do not, do some research and find out who it is you need to talk to at your insurance company should you have any questions. Establish a relationship with this person so they become familiar with your situation.

Insurance is an interesting labyrinth and truly requires a professional to navigate. Questions will come up concerning your deductible, which doctors are covered and which are not, how supplemental insurance works, how prescription deductibles work, when does one qualify for Medicare, and what is your next step? The list goes on and on. These are all very real, difficult questions that should be discussed with your insurance broker. Make this person your ally.

Helpful Tip #3: **How do you find an insurance broker?** It's as simple as opening up your local yellow pages or asking around. Word of mouth is a powerful tool, and as my broker says "good will travels a long way." Questions worth asking while you search for an insurance broker are:

1. How many years have you been working as a broker and are medical policies all you write?

   When looking for a broker, you want someone who specializes in medical insurance policies, not someone who dabbles in medical along with home and auto policies. You are looking for an advocate who knows how to navigate the web that is our medical system. You want a master of his or her trade, not a jack-of-all-trades.

2. If I have problems, questions or concerns, do I call the insurance company, or can I call you directly?

   The answer you are looking for is "please call me first and we will see if we can correct any issue you may be experiencing. If for some reason I do not have the correct answers, I (the broker) will help you contact the insurance company and fix the dilemma." By having a broker, you are looking for a knowledgeable individual who is willing to go to bat on your behalf.

3. Do you have support staff in your office should you (the broker) be away from the office or on vacation?

   There are two answers to this question; a simple "yes" or "no." Ideally, you would like to have support at all times, but I would not make this question a deal breaker. It is, however, helpful to know that there is staff available year round and that you are covered should you need help.

Helpful Tip #4: Are you aware that purchasing insurance online or on your own costs the same as having a broker write the policy on your behalf? There are several ways to receive coverage:

1. **If you are looking for an Individual Family Plan (IFP), you can go to the website of the company you believe will give you the best coverage and purchase a plan directly.**

   Different age groups tend to look for different features when purchasing insurance. Young adults swing toward low-cost plans, with low copayments and lower monthly dues because the chance of needing to use these plans are slim the younger and healthier you are. The younger generation is usually concerned with the cost of the individual doctor's visit because chances are they will not reach their deductible on a yearly basis. (I continue to say "chances" because having a less than ideal insurance plan can be a gamble you may win or lose.)

   As you get older, looking at the bottom line can be more beneficial. What is the maximum annual amount of out-of-pocket expense, including the deductible? This means once you have reached your deductible, how much more cost will you have to incur (per individual or as a family) before your insurance picks up 100 percent of the bill. Are you willing to do all this research on your own? Can you run the different scenarios and choose which plan is the correct for you? If this doesn't seem feasible, here is another option:

2. **Locate a respectable broker and have that individual find the correct plan to fit your needs.**

   As previously stated, the plans purchased through a broker cost the same as those purchased from the insurance company's website. The only extra investment on your part is time; the time it took to find and meet with your broker. The time you will save in the long run by having someone familiar with you, your family, and your situation could be priceless.

   If there is ever a question about how a certain billing has occurred, you have someone to call. If you are unsure if a practitioner is "in network," again, you have someone to call. If something catastrophic happens while on vacation in another country and you need to be reimbursed for expenses incurred, you now have someone who is willing to help you fill out the appropriate forms and recoup your losses.

   The major issues with Individual Family Plans occur if you are diagnosed with a condition and you do not have medical insurance at the time of diagnosis. The way medical insurance stands now, an IFP can deny coverage for preexisting conditions, making it very difficult to find coverage after a diagnosis is made.

3. **Group Plans can be obtained through an employer, and an individual cannot be denied coverage based on a preexisting condition.**
   Most policies require a six-month waiting period before coverage may begin. If you fit into this category and are unsure as to the specifics of your coverage, ask your employer or call your insurance company directly.

4. **U.S. Department of Veterans Affairs (VA).**
   The VA is a maze in and of itself that we will touch on very briefly. The VA is available to any person who served in active military duty and was released or discharged "under conditions other than dishonorable." Enrollment into the VA system, including more than 1,400 care sites, begins with an Application for Health Benefits. Not only does the VA offer medical care, they offer life insurance policies, burial, and memorial benefits as well as dependants and survivor health care. If you believe you or a loved one may qualify for VA benefits, educate yourself at www.va.gov or contact your local Veteran Affairs office.

5. **Medicare.**
   Medicare can be obtained one of two ways: an individual reaches sixty-five years of age, or an individual is under the age of sixty-five but has been collecting Social Security Disability Insurance (SSDI) for twenty-four months. Once one qualifies for Medicare, there are two parts; Part A covers hospital expenses, while Part B covers other medical expenses. Medicare Part A has a set deductible amount the patient must pay each time services are rendered at a hospital. Part B has a one-time set deductible amount. Once the deductible is met, a coinsurance of 20 percent of the billed amount will be billed to the individual.

   a. Supplemental insurance.
   This insurance can be an existing group coverage plan carried over from your employer or an IFP you keep as a supplemental, or you can purchase supplemental coverage from a number of insurance companies. Better yet, ask your broker which company and supplemental plan will work best for you. Supplemental insurance will cover the deductible for each hospital visit from Part A and the 20 percent coinsurance owed from Part B.
   When deciding on purchasing supplemental coverage, a number of variables should be considered. First, how old is the individual applying for the supplemental insurance? If the individual has qualified for Medicare be-

cause he or she is over the age of sixty-five, supplemental insurance can be quite affordable. If the individual is under the age of sixty-five and has qualified for Medicare based on SSDI, the supplemental insurance prices increase exponentially, so keeping one's preexisting insurance may be more cost effective.

b. The final option in this Medicare labyrinth is the Part D Prescription Drug Plan.

Part D plans, just like supplemental plans, are private companies contracted with Medicare and are completely separate entities from Part A and Part B. Different carriers approve or deny different medications and pharmacies. Medicare has created a database at www.medicare.gov/find-a-plan which allows each individual to type in their personal medications, pharmacy of choice, and zip code. The end result is a list of companies that not only cover your medications, but allow you to continue to use your pharmacy as well. Each company will show a breakdown of the retail price of your medication at the pharmacy of your choice, what your monthly premium will be if you choose their plan, what your deductible is, and finally what percentage of coinsurance you will pay. An example:

You are taking MagicMed and SleepPotion, you would like a thirty-day supply of each, and you would like to continue to use HappyDays Pharmacy. After filling out the questionnaire at Medicare.org, seventeen companies have come back offering you coverage. Company 1 says your medication costs $1,330.00–$1,470.00 retail on an annual basis, but with their coverage you will pay $14.90–$16.20 a month. Your deductible is $310, and once your deductible is met, your coinsurance is 20 percent, meaning you will pay about $2–$4 each time you need your meds. Being a quick thinker, you do the math and see that your medication will only cost you $31.10 a month with Company 1. After ten months, your deductible will be met and you will be paying an average of $6 a month (coinsurance) for the rest of the fiscal year, bringing your grand total to $335 a year for your two medications. Company 1 is offering this plan at a fee of $25.60 a month; a total of $307.20 in dues. Your annual dues ($307.20) plus the your out-of-pocket deductible and coinsurance ($335) cost a total of $642.20. Without this Part D plan you would be spending $2,800 retail for your medication. If you choose to go with Company 1, you will save $2,157.80.

If an IFP or a Group Plan has been carried over as a supplemental, this plan may already cover your medication and be far more cost effective. This is another example of how it can be beneficial to have a broker or benefits administrator from your employer.

Accountant/CPA

What is tax deductible? What is not? The list of questions for your CPA could be never ending, particularly if you are just beginning this journey. If you have an established relationship with your CPA, ask him or her to take some time to help you understand what it is that you should be tracking. Things you may never have considered tracking previously may now make all the difference. A few things you should consider tracking are:

1.   Any and all medical expenses, including, but not limited to:

•   Prescription Medication

•   All bills from physicians or medical facilities

•   Rented or purchased medical equipment, i.e., wheelchair, medical bed or walker

2.   Mileage to and from medical facilities.

•   *Recorded mileage can be written off at cents to the mile. The amount of cents per mile changes on an annual basis. Consult with your CPA to determine the amount of money per mile that is allotted for tax deduction.*

3.   Hotels you may have stayed in due to treatment out of area.

4.   Medical insurance premiums if self-employed.

Notary

As time progresses and documents pass through hands, there may be a time when notarization is required to authenticate or complete a document. A notary acts as a neutral party and witness to documents being signed.

Helpful Tip #5: Make sure the notary you establish a relationship with has the ability to travel. The time may come when the person needing to sign the documentation is unable to travel. Some hospitals have a notary on site.

End-of-Life Care

Have you discussed what your loved one's wishes are for his or her final days? Is being able to spend those final days at home a major concern? Do you understand the difference between palliative care and hospice? Do you have the resources to contact these establishments? End-of-life care may not seem relevant at this time; however, the truth is all of us, young or old, healthy or ill, should have this conversation with our families.

First and foremost, ask your doctors and treatment facility staff members for recommendations regarding the people to talk to about end-of-life care. There are usually social workers available to answer questions and point you in the correct direction.

Palliative care is different from hospice in that it is not end-of-life care. Palliative care can be utilized from the moment of the initial diagnosis, and it is intended, along with other treatments, to cure or prolong life. Hospice is usually brought in for end-of-life care, once curative treatments have been stopped. Both hospice and palliative care are designed to provide quality care through the disease progression. While palliative care helps manage symptoms and pain along with coordinating treatment, hospice is intended to keep the individual comfortable in the final months, weeks, or days of life.

Other Names and Numbers:

There are many other names and numbers you may find to be relevant and necessary to discuss. A few suggestions are:

Life and/or Long-Term Care Insurance: Does the patient have a life or long-term-care insurance policy? If so, what company carries the insurance policy, and is there a specific agent to contact should any questions arise?

Assisted-Living Facility: Depending upon your personal situation, an assisted-living facility may be the next step. How does the patient feel about residing in an assisted-living facility? Perhaps he or she already has a facility picked out!

Things to ask when looking into assisted-living facilities are, but not limited to:

- Who is the owner?
- What is the staff turnover?
- Does the facility have a Hospice Waiver?
- Is a vehicle available for residents' transportation?
- Take a look at the quality of life; how are the accommodations, food, and activities?
- When dealing with dementia, what level of dementia are they willing to care for? Do they have a locked ward?

Crematorium or Burial Facility: This may be a difficult name and number to write into this book. If you do not find it relevant, please pass this by. For many who require the assistance of this book, discussing this matter can be a bit of an elephant in the room. Know what your loved one's final wishes are. Would they like to be buried or cremated? Where would they like to be buried or have their ashes remain?

Helpful Tip #6: Know which establishment you would like to use and make prior arrangements. Once the end has come for the patient, you will know exactly who to call to help with the next step. These people will be very supportive and knowledgeable.

Name & Specialty

Make sure to write your doctor's or facility's full name. You will be surprised how many people share a last name or how many facilities end in "Imaging Center." Once you have the name written in, document your care provider's title or specialty. Is the provider a cardiologist, oncologist, radiologist, hematologist, neurologist, pathologist, anesthesiologist, pain management specialist, surgeon, psychiatrist, psychologist, speech therapist, occupational therapist, physical therapist, speech therapist, family therapist, or chiropractor? Do not exclude "alternative" options such as naturopath, certified massage therapist, or acupuncturist if these are modalities or treatments you choose to adopt.

Labs and facilities where you may have your blood work taken; a CT, PET scan, or MRI done; along with hospitals and pharmacies should be noted under "Name." Types of procedures/tests/treatments that are conducted at these particular locations or facilities may be documented under "Specialty."

For the remainder of the book, the term "facility" will be used to represent all centers, clinics, laboratories, hospitals, and other facilities. Every location a treatment, procedure, test, scan, or consultation is done should be in your phonebook, as well as the names of the doctors.

Phone Number

The availability of direct phone numbers to physicians and providers is limited. The phone number in this section is probably going to be the direct line to the front desk of your physician's office, pharmacy, or medical facility, or it may be to an answering service.

Helpful Tip #7: If the same individual picks up the phone day in and day out, make a little note of this person's name next to the phone number. Navigating the web of physicians' offices and facilities is all about establishing positive relationships.

Fax Number

The fax number is always a convenient number to have on hand in case you need to send a paper copy of a document. Some forms are still handwritten and are easily transferred from one facility to the next via fax. Nurses and other staff members will find the numbers they need to get the job done, but think of how quickly things can be expedited if you are organized and can immediately provide them with the information they need.

E-Mail

An increasing number of physicians are relying on e-mail to communicate with patients and other facilities. Check the business card of your physician and see if there is an e-mail contact available. Add this contact to your phone book section for safe keeping.

Helpful Tip #8: If there is an e-mail address on your physician's business card, ask your physician if he or she would prefer you contact them via e-mail for questions.

Address

When writing in the address of your physician or medical facility, make sure to document the correct suite or floor. Addresses will come in handy when you are working with several physicians or specialists within different facilities. You may be working with facilities in different cities or even states. Again, the staff of any office will eventually find the contact information they need to send off documents or request results from a separate facility. The goal is to be able to provide them with this information to limit delays.

Helpful Tip #9: When working with a facility or physician from out of your town, having the address to your local pharmacy handy will be a big help. If a prescription needs to be called or faxed in, you will have the correct address (so your medications do not go to the pharmacy on the other side of town with the same name).

Contact Name & Contact Number

Nine times out of ten, this section will be used for a nurse or physician's assistant (PA) in your physician's office. This individual should be at the top of your list of people with whom you want to establish a working relationship. This is usually the person you will talk to when you have a concern or need just about anything. If the nurse or assistant is unable to rectify the situation, he or she will be able to steer you in the right direction. Also this individual usually will have a direct line, so you can by-pass the nice person at the front desk.

Others who may end up in this box would be the pharmacist, the technician at the pharmacy who runs the prescriptions through insurance, or any individual with whom you have frequent interactions.

NAME	
SPECIALTY	
PHONE	FAX
EMAIL	
ADDRESS	
CONTACT NAME	
CONTACT NUMBER	

NAME	
SPECIALTY	
PHONE	FAX
EMAIL	
ADDRESS	
CONTACT NAME	
CONTACT NUMBER	

NAME	
SPECIALTY	
PHONE	FAX
EMAIL	
ADDRESS	
CONTACT NAME	
CONTACT NUMBER	

NAME

SPECIALTY

PHONE | FAX

EMAIL

ADDRESS

CONTACT NAME

CONTACT NUMBER

NAME

SPECIALTY

PHONE | FAX

EMAIL

ADDRESS

CONTACT NAME

CONTACT NUMBER

NAME

SPECIALTY

PHONE | FAX

EMAIL

ADDRESS

CONTACT NAME

CONTACT NUMBER

NAME	
SPECIALTY	
PHONE	FAX
EMAIL	
ADDRESS	
CONTACT NAME	
CONTACT NUMBER	

NAME	
SPECIALTY	
PHONE	FAX
EMAIL	
ADDRESS	
CONTACT NAME	
CONTACT NUMBER	

NAME	
SPECIALTY	
PHONE	FAX
EMAIL	
ADDRESS	
CONTACT NAME	
CONTACT NUMBER	

NAME

SPECIALTY

PHONE

FAX

EMAIL

ADDRESS

CONTACT NAME

CONTACT NUMBER

NAME

SPECIALTY

PHONE

FAX

EMAIL

ADDRESS

CONTACT NAME

CONTACT NUMBER

NAME

SPECIALTY

PHONE

FAX

EMAIL

ADDRESS

CONTACT NAME

CONTACT NUMBER

NAME

SPECIALTY

PHONE | FAX

EMAIL

ADDRESS

CONTACT NAME

CONTACT NUMBER

NAME

SPECIALTY

PHONE | FAX

EMAIL

ADDRESS

CONTACT NAME

CONTACT NUMBER

NAME

SPECIALTY

PHONE | FAX

EMAIL

ADDRESS

CONTACT NAME

CONTACT NUMBER

NAME	
SPECIALTY	
PHONE	FAX
EMAIL	
ADDRESS	
CONTACT NAME	
CONTACT NUMBER	

NAME	
SPECIALTY	
PHONE	FAX
EMAIL	
ADDRESS	
CONTACT NAME	
CONTACT NUMBER	

NAME	
SPECIALTY	
PHONE	FAX
EMAIL	
ADDRESS	
CONTACT NAME	
CONTACT NUMBER	

NAME	
SPECIALTY	
PHONE	FAX
EMAIL	
ADDRESS	
CONTACT NAME	
CONTACT NUMBER	

NAME	
SPECIALTY	
PHONE	FAX
EMAIL	
ADDRESS	
CONTACT NAME	
CONTACT NUMBER	

NAME	
SPECIALTY	
PHONE	FAX
EMAIL	
ADDRESS	
CONTACT NAME	
CONTACT NUMBER	

NAME

SPECIALTY

PHONE | FAX

EMAIL

ADDRESS

CONTACT NAME

CONTACT NUMBER

NAME

SPECIALTY

PHONE | FAX

EMAIL

ADDRESS

CONTACT NAME

CONTACT NUMBER

NAME

SPECIALTY

PHONE | FAX

EMAIL

ADDRESS

CONTACT NAME

CONTACT NUMBER

NAME	
SPECIALTY	
PHONE	FAX
EMAIL	
ADDRESS	
CONTACT NAME	
CONTACT NUMBER	

NAME	
SPECIALTY	
PHONE	FAX
EMAIL	
ADDRESS	
CONTACT NAME	
CONTACT NUMBER	

NAME	
SPECIALTY	
PHONE	FAX
EMAIL	
ADDRESS	
CONTACT NAME	
CONTACT NUMBER	

NAME

SPECIALTY

PHONE	FAX

EMAIL

ADDRESS

CONTACT NAME

CONTACT NUMBER

NAME

SPECIALTY

PHONE	FAX

EMAIL

ADDRESS

CONTACT NAME

CONTACT NUMBER

NAME

SPECIALTY

PHONE	FAX

EMAIL

ADDRESS

CONTACT NAME

CONTACT NUMBER

NAME	
SPECIALTY	
PHONE	FAX
EMAIL	
ADDRESS	
CONTACT NAME	
CONTACT NUMBER	

NAME	
SPECIALTY	
PHONE	FAX
EMAIL	
ADDRESS	
CONTACT NAME	
CONTACT NUMBER	

NAME	
SPECIALTY	
PHONE	FAX
EMAIL	
ADDRESS	
CONTACT NAME	
CONTACT NUMBER	

Medication & Supplement Breakdown

Each section of this book is important and requires time and attention to keep up-to-date. The Medication section may be the most important to keep organized. Medications change, doses change, frequencies change. Tracking these changes does not need to be a practice in memorization. Eventually something will slip through the cracks if it is not written down. Below is a diagram of a prescription label that will help you fill in the following section.

HappyDays Pharmacy **(555)555-5555**
1234 Smile Lane · Date Filled: 01/01/2012
Your Town, CA 95555
12345 987654
Smith, Victoria
333 Fern Street (555) 565-6565
Your Town, CA 95555
TAKE 1 TO 2 TABLETS BY MOUTH EVERY 4 HOURS
AS NEEDED FOR PAIN.
MagicMed 5mg
Generic for ElixerPlus
Oblong purple
Pr. JOHN, DOE D (555)565-1234
DISCARD AFTER 01/01/2012
NO REFILLS LEFT QTY 80

Start Date

The start date of the medication is the date you first began the medication. This date will not change. It does not refer to the date that any particular bottle was picked up from the pharmacy, but only to the first time you began the medication.

Medication Name

What is the name of the medication? As you see on the diagram on the previous page, there is the name of the medication, possibly followed by "generic for" and then another name for the medication. If the medication is a generic, check the small box inside this square. Write out the full name of the medications, for example: *MagicMed 5mg generic for ElixerPlus.*

Description

Below the name of the medication on the prescription label are usually a few words describing what the medication looks like: "Round light blue" or "Oval white with black stripe." Write this description down so you have an idea of what this pill should look like. The time may come that prescriptions are being taken every few hours, seven days a week. It is common to divide a week's worth of medication into a pill dispenser, divided into Early AM, Mid AM, Noon, Early PM, and Late PM. Having an idea of what each pill looks like and double confirming that the correct medication is being taken at the correct time is very important to the safety and well-being of the individual.

Purpose

Why is this medication or supplement being prescribed or suggested? There are usually a few sentences describing how to take the medication in the center of the label, followed by "for _____." This could be "for pain," "for depression," "for anxiety," "for nausea," or any number of ailments. Make a quick note of the purpose of this medication, vitamin, or supplement.

Prescribing Physician

As seen in the previous diagram, the prescribing physician's name is usually located under the medication name, along with the physician's contact information. You only need to write in the name of the physician, as you should have all of this individual's contact information in your phone book.

Some prescriptions are written with several refills on one slip, while others are a triplicate and require a new prescription for every refill. Knowing which physician to call to request a prescription refill will expedite the process.

Quick Vocab Lesson: Triplicate (in reference to prescription forms). When prescribing a Schedule II drug, a physician must write out a "triplicate" prescription. The prescribing physician will keep one copy of the triplicate for his or her records, the pharmacy will keep one copy, and the designated state agency will keep the third copy. The program was designed as a check to control Schedule II drugs. It helps track the patient's use of the substance and the physician's prescribing practices, and thus it helps deter the controlled substances from making it to the "streets" to be sold illegally. It is common for medications requiring a triplicate to not be prescribed with automatic refills. A new prescription must be written by a prescribing physician each time a refill is required.

Prescription Number

The prescription number is commonly found in the upper-right- or left-hand corner (depending upon your pharmacy). This number correlates directly to you and one specific medication, and it can be particularly helpful if you have a prescription that has several refills available. Most pharmacies offer a "call-in" database. When you are close to running out of a prescription, you can call in, key in your prescription number, confirm the name of the medication, and voila! Your medication will be ready in the next few hours for pickup.

Pharmacy

As stated earlier, you may be working with more than one pharmacy, depending upon the types of prescriptions you are filling. Making a quick note of which pharmacy provides each medication will help keep you organized. You would hate to wait in line at one pharmacy, only to finally make it to the counter and realize you are at the incorrect pharmacy. The pharmacy's address and contact information will be on the medication label, but it should also be in your phone book.

Dose and Frequency

How many of each pill or how many cc's/tablespoons will you be needing of each medication? How often will the medication be given? If the medication is in pill form, we know the potency of the medication because that information was already documented in the "Medication Name" box of this section. As in the previous diagram, we know the medication is MagicMed 5mg generic for ElixerPlus. In the center of the label, the directions say TAKE 1 TO 2 TABLETS BY MOUTH EVERY 4 HOURS AS NEEDED FOR PAIN. "1 tablet" or "5mg" is our "dose" in this case. In the dose box, write "5mg." "Every four hours" is our "frequency." Some medications may state "3 times daily," "Every 48 hours" or "As needed." If you need clarification, take a moment to ask your pharmacist or physician until you fully understand how each medication should be taken.

Discontinue Date (D/C)

Knowing when you stopped taking a medication can be equally as important as knowing the start date. Some medications cannot be taken within a certain length of time after another. Having all the information helps paint a clear picture of the progression and changes you have made throughout the process.

Side Effects

Each prescription has a list of possible side effects. These are only possibilities and the patient may experience none or all of them. Take a moment to write in the side effects the patient does experience after taking a particular medication. Having an understanding of which medication is creating which side effects can better help the prescribing physician find the appropriate balance and combination of medications.

START DATE	D/C	MEDICATION	☐ GENERIC
DOSE	FREQUENCY	PHARMACY	Rx
DESCRIPTION			Rx PHYSICIAN
SIDE EFFECTS			PURPOSE

START DATE	D/C	MEDICATION	☐ GENERIC
DOSE	FREQUENCY	PHARMACY	Rx
DESCRIPTION			Rx PHYSICIAN
SIDE EFFECTS			PURPOSE

START DATE	D/C	MEDICATION	☐ GENERIC
DOSE	FREQUENCY	PHARMACY	Rx
DESCRIPTION			Rx PHYSICIAN
SIDE EFFECTS			PURPOSE

START DATE	D/C	MEDICATION	☐ GENERIC
DOSE	FREQUENCY	PHARMACY	Rx
DESCRIPTION			Rx PHYSICIAN
SIDE EFFECTS			PURPOSE

START DATE	D/C	MEDICATION	☐ GENERIC
DOSE	FREQUENCY	PHARMACY	Rx
DESCRIPTION			Rx PHYSICIAN
SIDE EFFECTS			PURPOSE

START DATE	D/C	MEDICATION	☐ GENERIC
DOSE	FREQUENCY	PHARMACY	Rx
DESCRIPTION			Rx PHYSICIAN
SIDE EFFECTS			PURPOSE

START DATE	D/C	MEDICATION		☐ GENERIC
DOSE	FREQUENCY	PHARMACY		Rx
DESCRIPTION			Rx PHYSICIAN	
SIDE EFFECTS			PURPOSE	

START DATE	D/C	MEDICATION		☐ GENERIC
DOSE	FREQUENCY	PHARMACY		Rx
DESCRIPTION			Rx PHYSICIAN	
SIDE EFFECTS			PURPOSE	

START DATE	D/C	MEDICATION		☐ GENERIC
DOSE	FREQUENCY	PHARMACY		Rx
DESCRIPTION			Rx PHYSICIAN	
SIDE EFFECTS			PURPOSE	

START DATE	D/C	MEDICATION		☐ GENERIC
DOSE	FREQUENCY	PHARMACY		Rx
DESCRIPTION			Rx PHYSICIAN	
SIDE EFFECTS			PURPOSE	

START DATE	D/C	MEDICATION		☐ GENERIC
DOSE	FREQUENCY	PHARMACY		Rx
DESCRIPTION			Rx PHYSICIAN	
SIDE EFFECTS			PURPOSE	

START DATE	D/C	MEDICATION		☐ GENERIC
DOSE	FREQUENCY	PHARMACY		Rx
DESCRIPTION			Rx PHYSICIAN	
SIDE EFFECTS			PURPOSE	

START DATE	D/C	MEDICATION		☐ GENERIC
DOSE	FREQUENCY	PHARMACY		Rx
DESCRIPTION			Rx PHYSICIAN	
SIDE EFFECTS			PURPOSE	

START DATE	D/C	MEDICATION		☐ GENERIC
DOSE	FREQUENCY	PHARMACY		Rx
DESCRIPTION			Rx PHYSICIAN	
SIDE EFFECTS			PURPOSE	

START DATE	D/C	MEDICATION		☐ GENERIC
DOSE	FREQUENCY	PHARMACY		Rx
DESCRIPTION			Rx PHYSICIAN	
SIDE EFFECTS			PURPOSE	

START DATE	D/C	MEDICATION		☐ GENERIC
DOSE	FREQUENCY	PHARMACY		Rx
DESCRIPTION			Rx PHYSICIAN	
SIDE EFFECTS			PURPOSE	

START DATE	D/C	MEDICATION		☐ GENERIC
DOSE	FREQUENCY	PHARMACY		Rx
DESCRIPTION			Rx PHYSICIAN	
SIDE EFFECTS			PURPOSE	

START DATE	D/C	MEDICATION		☐ GENERIC
DOSE	FREQUENCY	PHARMACY		Rx
DESCRIPTION			Rx PHYSICIAN	
SIDE EFFECTS			PURPOSE	

START DATE	D/C	MEDICATION		☐ GENERIC
DOSE	FREQUENCY	PHARMACY		Rx
DESCRIPTION			Rx PHYSICIAN	
SIDE EFFECTS			PURPOSE	

START DATE	D/C	MEDICATION		☐ GENERIC
DOSE	FREQUENCY	PHARMACY		Rx
DESCRIPTION			Rx PHYSICIAN	
SIDE EFFECTS			PURPOSE	

START DATE	D/C	MEDICATION		☐ GENERIC
DOSE	FREQUENCY	PHARMACY		Rx
DESCRIPTION			Rx PHYSICIAN	
SIDE EFFECTS			PURPOSE	

START DATE	D/C	MEDICATION		☐ GENERIC
DOSE	FREQUENCY	PHARMACY		Rx
DESCRIPTION			Rx PHYSICIAN	
SIDE EFFECTS			PURPOSE	

START DATE	D/C	MEDICATION		☐ GENERIC
DOSE	FREQUENCY	PHARMACY		Rx
DESCRIPTION			Rx PHYSICIAN	
SIDE EFFECTS			PURPOSE	

START DATE	D/C	MEDICATION		☐ GENERIC
DOSE	FREQUENCY	PHARMACY		Rx
DESCRIPTION			Rx PHYSICIAN	
SIDE EFFECTS			PURPOSE	

START DATE	D/C	MEDICATION	☐ GENERIC
DOSE	FREQUENCY	PHARMACY	Rx
DESCRIPTION			Rx PHYSICIAN
SIDE EFFECTS			PURPOSE

START DATE	D/C	MEDICATION	☐ GENERIC
DOSE	FREQUENCY	PHARMACY	Rx
DESCRIPTION			Rx PHYSICIAN
SIDE EFFECTS			PURPOSE

START DATE	D/C	MEDICATION	☐ GENERIC
DOSE	FREQUENCY	PHARMACY	Rx
DESCRIPTION			Rx PHYSICIAN
SIDE EFFECTS			PURPOSE

START DATE	D/C	MEDICATION	☐ GENERIC
DOSE	FREQUENCY	PHARMACY	Rx
DESCRIPTION			Rx PHYSICIAN
SIDE EFFECTS			PURPOSE

START DATE	D/C	MEDICATION	☐ GENERIC
DOSE	FREQUENCY	PHARMACY	Rx
DESCRIPTION			Rx PHYSICIAN
SIDE EFFECTS			PURPOSE

START DATE	D/C	MEDICATION	☐ GENERIC
DOSE	FREQUENCY	PHARMACY	Rx
DESCRIPTION			Rx PHYSICIAN
SIDE EFFECTS			PURPOSE

START DATE	D/C	MEDICATION	☐ GENERIC

DOSE	FREQUENCY	PHARMACY	Rx

DESCRIPTION	Rx PHYSICIAN
SIDE EFFECTS	PURPOSE

START DATE	D/C	MEDICATION	☐ GENERIC

DOSE	FREQUENCY	PHARMACY	Rx

DESCRIPTION	Rx PHYSICIAN
SIDE EFFECTS	PURPOSE

START DATE	D/C	MEDICATION	☐ GENERIC

DOSE	FREQUENCY	PHARMACY	Rx

DESCRIPTION	Rx PHYSICIAN
SIDE EFFECTS	PURPOSE

START DATE	D/C	MEDICATION	☐ GENERIC

DOSE	FREQUENCY	PHARMACY	Rx

DESCRIPTION	Rx PHYSICIAN
SIDE EFFECTS	PURPOSE

START DATE	D/C	MEDICATION	☐ GENERIC

DOSE	FREQUENCY	PHARMACY	Rx

DESCRIPTION	Rx PHYSICIAN
SIDE EFFECTS	PURPOSE

START DATE	D/C	MEDICATION	☐ GENERIC

DOSE	FREQUENCY	PHARMACY	Rx

DESCRIPTION	Rx PHYSICIAN
SIDE EFFECTS	PURPOSE

START DATE	D/C	MEDICATION	☐ GENERIC
DOSE	FREQUENCY	PHARMACY	Rx
DESCRIPTION			Rx PHYSICIAN
SIDE EFFECTS			PURPOSE

START DATE	D/C	MEDICATION	☐ GENERIC
DOSE	FREQUENCY	PHARMACY	Rx
DESCRIPTION			Rx PHYSICIAN
SIDE EFFECTS			PURPOSE

START DATE	D/C	MEDICATION	☐ GENERIC
DOSE	FREQUENCY	PHARMACY	Rx
DESCRIPTION			Rx PHYSICIAN
SIDE EFFECTS			PURPOSE

START DATE	D/C	MEDICATION	☐ GENERIC
DOSE	FREQUENCY	PHARMACY	Rx
DESCRIPTION			Rx PHYSICIAN
SIDE EFFECTS			PURPOSE

START DATE	D/C	MEDICATION	☐ GENERIC
DOSE	FREQUENCY	PHARMACY	Rx
DESCRIPTION			Rx PHYSICIAN
SIDE EFFECTS			PURPOSE

START DATE	D/C	MEDICATION	☐ GENERIC
DOSE	FREQUENCY	PHARMACY	Rx
DESCRIPTION			Rx PHYSICIAN
SIDE EFFECTS			PURPOSE

START DATE	D/C	MEDICATION		☐ GENERIC
DOSE	FREQUENCY	PHARMACY		Rx
DESCRIPTION			Rx PHYSICIAN	
SIDE EFFECTS			PURPOSE	

START DATE	D/C	MEDICATION		☐ GENERIC
DOSE	FREQUENCY	PHARMACY		Rx
DESCRIPTION			Rx PHYSICIAN	
SIDE EFFECTS			PURPOSE	

START DATE	D/C	MEDICATION		☐ GENERIC
DOSE	FREQUENCY	PHARMACY		Rx
DESCRIPTION			Rx PHYSICIAN	
SIDE EFFECTS			PURPOSE	

START DATE	D/C	MEDICATION		☐ GENERIC
DOSE	FREQUENCY	PHARMACY		Rx
DESCRIPTION			Rx PHYSICIAN	
SIDE EFFECTS			PURPOSE	

START DATE	D/C	MEDICATION		☐ GENERIC
DOSE	FREQUENCY	PHARMACY		Rx
DESCRIPTION			Rx PHYSICIAN	
SIDE EFFECTS			PURPOSE	

START DATE	D/C	MEDICATION		☐ GENERIC
DOSE	FREQUENCY	PHARMACY		Rx
DESCRIPTION			Rx PHYSICIAN	
SIDE EFFECTS			PURPOSE	

START DATE	D/C	MEDICATION		☐ GENERIC
DOSE	FREQUENCY	PHARMACY		Rx
DESCRIPTION			Rx PHYSICIAN	
SIDE EFFECTS			PURPOSE	

START DATE	D/C	MEDICATION		☐ GENERIC
DOSE	FREQUENCY	PHARMACY		Rx
DESCRIPTION			Rx PHYSICIAN	
SIDE EFFECTS			PURPOSE	

START DATE	D/C	MEDICATION		☐ GENERIC
DOSE	FREQUENCY	PHARMACY		Rx
DESCRIPTION			Rx PHYSICIAN	
SIDE EFFECTS			PURPOSE	

START DATE	D/C	MEDICATION		☐ GENERIC
DOSE	FREQUENCY	PHARMACY		Rx
DESCRIPTION			Rx PHYSICIAN	
SIDE EFFECTS			PURPOSE	

START DATE	D/C	MEDICATION		☐ GENERIC
DOSE	FREQUENCY	PHARMACY		Rx
DESCRIPTION			Rx PHYSICIAN	
SIDE EFFECTS			PURPOSE	

START DATE	D/C	MEDICATION		☐ GENERIC
DOSE	FREQUENCY	PHARMACY		Rx
DESCRIPTION			Rx PHYSICIAN	
SIDE EFFECTS			PURPOSE	

START DATE	D/C	MEDICATION	☐ GENERIC
DOSE	FREQUENCY	PHARMACY	Rx
DESCRIPTION		Rx PHYSICIAN	
SIDE EFFECTS		PURPOSE	

START DATE	D/C	MEDICATION	☐ GENERIC
DOSE	FREQUENCY	PHARMACY	Rx
DESCRIPTION		Rx PHYSICIAN	
SIDE EFFECTS		PURPOSE	

START DATE	D/C	MEDICATION	☐ GENERIC
DOSE	FREQUENCY	PHARMACY	Rx
DESCRIPTION		Rx PHYSICIAN	
SIDE EFFECTS		PURPOSE	

START DATE	D/C	MEDICATION	☐ GENERIC
DOSE	FREQUENCY	PHARMACY	Rx
DESCRIPTION		Rx PHYSICIAN	
SIDE EFFECTS		PURPOSE	

START DATE	D/C	MEDICATION	☐ GENERIC
DOSE	FREQUENCY	PHARMACY	Rx
DESCRIPTION		Rx PHYSICIAN	
SIDE EFFECTS		PURPOSE	

START DATE	D/C	MEDICATION	☐ GENERIC
DOSE	FREQUENCY	PHARMACY	Rx
DESCRIPTION		Rx PHYSICIAN	
SIDE EFFECTS		PURPOSE	

START DATE	D/C	MEDICATION		☐ GENERIC
DOSE	FREQUENCY	PHARMACY		Rx
DESCRIPTION			Rx PHYSICIAN	
SIDE EFFECTS			PURPOSE	

START DATE	D/C	MEDICATION		☐ GENERIC
DOSE	FREQUENCY	PHARMACY		Rx
DESCRIPTION			Rx PHYSICIAN	
SIDE EFFECTS			PURPOSE	

START DATE	D/C	MEDICATION		☐ GENERIC
DOSE	FREQUENCY	PHARMACY		Rx
DESCRIPTION			Rx PHYSICIAN	
SIDE EFFECTS			PURPOSE	

START DATE	D/C	MEDICATION		☐ GENERIC
DOSE	FREQUENCY	PHARMACY		Rx
DESCRIPTION			Rx PHYSICIAN	
SIDE EFFECTS			PURPOSE	

START DATE	D/C	MEDICATION		☐ GENERIC
DOSE	FREQUENCY	PHARMACY		Rx
DESCRIPTION			Rx PHYSICIAN	
SIDE EFFECTS			PURPOSE	

START DATE	D/C	MEDICATION		☐ GENERIC
DOSE	FREQUENCY	PHARMACY		Rx
DESCRIPTION			Rx PHYSICIAN	
SIDE EFFECTS			PURPOSE	

START DATE	D/C	MEDICATION	☐ GENERIC
DOSE	FREQUENCY	PHARMACY	Rx
DESCRIPTION		Rx PHYSICIAN	
SIDE EFFECTS		PURPOSE	

START DATE	D/C	MEDICATION	☐ GENERIC
DOSE	FREQUENCY	PHARMACY	Rx
DESCRIPTION		Rx PHYSICIAN	
SIDE EFFECTS		PURPOSE	

START DATE	D/C	MEDICATION	☐ GENERIC
DOSE	FREQUENCY	PHARMACY	Rx
DESCRIPTION		Rx PHYSICIAN	
SIDE EFFECTS		PURPOSE	

START DATE	D/C	MEDICATION	☐ GENERIC
DOSE	FREQUENCY	PHARMACY	Rx
DESCRIPTION		Rx PHYSICIAN	
SIDE EFFECTS		PURPOSE	

START DATE	D/C	MEDICATION	☐ GENERIC
DOSE	FREQUENCY	PHARMACY	Rx
DESCRIPTION		Rx PHYSICIAN	
SIDE EFFECTS		PURPOSE	

START DATE	D/C	MEDICATION	☐ GENERIC
DOSE	FREQUENCY	PHARMACY	Rx
DESCRIPTION		Rx PHYSICIAN	
SIDE EFFECTS		PURPOSE	

Medication Pickup Chart

The more hands involved in dropping off and picking up prescriptions, as well as distributing medications, the larger the opportunity for things to go awry. This subsection is designed to help you track "who," "what," and "where."

Date

What is the date the prescription was picked up? This date is helpful for several reasons. Prescriptions are usually given in thirty-day increments. As more and more medications are prescribed, it becomes harder to keep track of when each prescription is eligible for refill. It would be nice if the medications were on a cycle that required one monthly trip to the pharmacy; unfortunately, this will rarely be the case.

Medication

What is the name of the medication? Use the brand name or the generic name. If you are not sure whether the prescription is generic or brand (hydrocodon vs. Norco), ask your pharmacist.

Caregiver

Who is the person who picked up this prescription? If there are any special instructions, this is the person to ask. If you are the caregiver picking up the medication and you have questions, don't be shy; the pharmacist will always take a moment to answer your questions.

Pharmacy

From which pharmacy was this medication picked up? Ideally, you would like to use the same pharmacy for all of your prescriptions. However, depending on the schedule of the drug, some pharmacies may not keep a particular medication in stock, meaning you may need to use multiple pharmacies to begin with. Usually, once the "trial-and-error" period is over and a suitable combination of medications is found, your pharmacy will be happy to carry what you need or order it in a timely fashion. In the meantime, keeping track of which pharmacy is distributing each medication will help with tracking and organization. Consider your choice of pharmacies. Do they have a drive through? Is there a 24-hour window?

Quick Vocab Lesson: Schedule (in reference to drugs). Prescription drugs are divided into classes, then into Schedules, I, II, III, IV, and V. Schedules were designed to rate drugs on their potential for abuse and medical relevance. The lowest number (I) has the highest potential for abuse and no medical relevance. A Schedule II drug has proven medical relevance but a high potential for abuse and dependence. The Schedules work all the way to V, which has the lowest potential for abuse, such as cough syrup.

Payment Method

How was the prescription purchased? Was a check written, an ATM card swiped, or cash exchanged? Why does it matter how the prescription was purchased, as long as the patient gets what they need, you ask? This is another way of tracking the medications and their cost. Prescription medications are tax deductible, and at this point I'm sure you would like to get as many deductions as possible. That's another reason to have a CPA's number in the personal information section of this book.

Helpful Tip #10: If the patient you are caring for does not already have a medical bank account, consider opening one. Place a sum of money in the account and purchase all medically relevant material out of this account. All copayments, medical bills, equipment, and prescriptions should be paid from the same account. This will allow you to have a more accurate record of all medical expenses. At the end of the year, your CPA should be able to help you with what is and is not tax deductible.

Amount

How much was the medication? If you swiped an ATM card or wrote a check, did you document the amount in the account register? You may have forgotten to record the amount in your account register, but you will still have a record of the transaction if you record it in this section. Again, everything here is designed to cross reference and intercept any miscommunication or errors. Let's say you picked up the medication on January 11 and it cost $12.33. On February 10, Uncle Joe picked the medication up and it cost $96.00. Did the insurance not go through? Was Uncle Joe not given a generic brand this time? Because of this documentation system, a red flag has been thrown up and attention has been brought to the situation.

Helpful Tip #11: There may be times when the pharmacy itself is out of a certain medication. You may pay for it in full, but only receive a ten- or twelve-day supply. Make a note in this section that the prescription has been paid in full but the second half must be picked up on date XX/XX/XXXX.

DATE	MEDICATION	CAREGIVER	PHARMACY	PAYMENT METHOD	AMOUNT
1/11/2012	MagicMed	Susie	Happy Days Pharmacy	Med ATM	12.33
1/12/2012	SleepPotion	Nick	Happy Days Pharmacy	Med Check #1234	17.97
Pharmacy only had half of prescription avail. Should be filled by 14th. Paid in full				
1/14/2012	SleepPotion	Susie	Happy Days Pharmacy	Paid 1/12/2012	0.00

DATE	MEDICATION	CAREGIVER	PHARMACY	PAYMENT METHOD	AMOUNT

Medication Pickup Chart

DATE	MEDICATION	CAREGIVER	PHARMACY	PAYMENT METHOD	AMOUNT

DATE	MEDICATION	CAREGIVER	PHARMACY	PAYMENT METHOD	AMOUNT

Medication Pickup Chart

DATE	MEDICATION	CAREGIVER	PHARMACY	PAYMENT METHOD	AMOUNT

DATE	MEDICATION	CAREGIVER	PHARMACY	PAYMENT METHOD	AMOUNT

Medication Pickup Chart

DATE	MEDICATION	CAREGIVER	PHARMACY	PAYMENT METHOD	AMOUNT

DATE	MEDICATION	CAREGIVER	PHARMACY	PAYMENT METHOD	AMOUNT

Physician

Which physician are you going to see? This section is to be used for appointments with physicians, not for scans or treatment appointments. Scans, tests, procedures, and treatments have a section of their own coming up.

Is this physician in your phone book? If not, make sure to put his/her information in the phone book because you now have an established relationship with this provider.

Date & Time

This may seem unimportant. But this book is all about documentation that allows you to look back and keep everything organized and in perspective. Having dates and times will help you in the long run track the progression of the disease or disorder. It will keep all the caregivers organized, as everyone will have access to this information. It will also help you come up with a schedule to best suit the patient's needs.

What if you begin to notice that the person you are caring for is awfully tired or distracted during a visit to Dr. Smith, but is very focused every time you see Dr. Jones? Take a look at your appointment sheets. Are there any patterns? Perhaps Dr. Smith's appointments are always at 2 PM, right after the patient takes a dose of afternoon medication. Dr. Jones's appointments are at 10 AM after a nice hardy breakfast. So what do you do about this predicament? Change Dr. Smith's appointment time? Can the medication wait until after Dr. Smith's appointment? Use this section to find patterns that precipitate best care.

Caregiver

Which caregiver is slated to take the patient to this appointment? Have this caretaker information filled out in advanced. Remember, this booklet stays with the individual who is sick, allowing whoever is acting as caregiver to have full knowledge of the medical care and history. This will also allow the next caregiver to know who to ask if they have questions about the last appointment or what to expect from the next appointment.

Results/Outcome

What occurred at this appointment? Was a test/scan/procedure prescribed or referred? Was medication changed? Were the results of a previous test/scan/procedure discussed? What is the next step?

Include any information that seems relevant to this particular appointment. If you are unsure if something is relevant, write it in. This will be useful information to bring back and share with the other individuals aiding in the caring process.

Helpful Tip 12: If possible, bring more than one person to any given appointment. Every person hears something different when discussing information with physicians or medical providers. This entire situation can be stressful. You are being exposed to a whole new language. Having extra ears will increase your chances of getting the most knowledge out of any given appointment.

Next Appointment Date

Did you reschedule with this physician when you left the appointment? This new appointment date and time should be in this box, as well as in your 52-week day planner provided at the back of this book. If possible, when you get back to "home base," designate who will be responsible for taking the individual to this follow-up appointment.

Purpose

Now that you have scheduled a next appointment, what is the purpose? If a scan or test was prescribed, will the results be in next time? If a medication was changed, would the physician like a follow-up report of side effects? Take a moment and write a small note about what is to occur at the next appointment, in case you are not the caregiver who is going to be attending. This way, whoever ends up taking the patient to his or her next appointment will be up to speed and informed about what is to occur.

Physicians do the best they can, but we all know how busy they can be. It is not uncommon to go to an appointment expecting to get the results of a scan and they are completely overlooked. Be informed and know why you are there.

DATE	PHYSICIAN
TIME	CAREGIVER
RESULTS	
NEXT APP. DATE	PURPOSE

DATE	PHYSICIAN
TIME	CAREGIVER
RESULTS	
NEXT APP. DATE	PURPOSE

DATE	PHYSICIAN
TIME	CAREGIVER
RESULTS	
NEXT APP. DATE	PURPOSE

DATE	PHYSICIAN
TIME	CAREGIVER
RESULTS	
NEXT APP. DATE	PURPOSE

DATE	PHYSICIAN
TIME	CAREGIVER
RESULTS	
NEXT APP. DATE	PURPOSE

DATE	PHYSICIAN	
TIME	CAREGIVER	
RESULTS		
NEXT APP. DATE	PURPOSE	

DATE	PHYSICIAN	
TIME	CAREGIVER	
RESULTS		
NEXT APP. DATE	PURPOSE	

DATE	PHYSICIAN	
TIME	CAREGIVER	
RESULTS		
NEXT APP. DATE	PURPOSE	

DATE	PHYSICIAN	
TIME	CAREGIVER	
RESULTS		
NEXT APP. DATE	PURPOSE	

DATE	PHYSICIAN	
TIME	CAREGIVER	
RESULTS		
NEXT APP. DATE	PURPOSE	

DATE	PHYSICIAN
TIME	CAREGIVER
RESULTS	
NEXT APP. DATE	PURPOSE

DATE	PHYSICIAN
TIME	CAREGIVER
RESULTS	
NEXT APP. DATE	PURPOSE

DATE	PHYSICIAN
TIME	CAREGIVER
RESULTS	
NEXT APP. DATE	PURPOSE

DATE	PHYSICIAN
TIME	CAREGIVER
RESULTS	
NEXT APP. DATE	PURPOSE

DATE	PHYSICIAN
TIME	CAREGIVER
RESULTS	
NEXT APP. DATE	PURPOSE

DATE	PHYSICIAN
TIME	CAREGIVER
RESULTS	
NEXT APP. DATE	PURPOSE

DATE	PHYSICIAN
TIME	CAREGIVER
RESULTS	
NEXT APP. DATE	PURPOSE

DATE	PHYSICIAN
TIME	CAREGIVER
RESULTS	
NEXT APP. DATE	PURPOSE

DATE	PHYSICIAN
TIME	CAREGIVER
RESULTS	
NEXT APP. DATE	PURPOSE

DATE	PHYSICIAN
TIME	CAREGIVER
RESULTS	
NEXT APP. DATE	PURPOSE

DATE	PHYSICIAN
TIME	CAREGIVER
RESULTS	
NEXT APP. DATE	PURPOSE

DATE	PHYSICIAN
TIME	CAREGIVER
RESULTS	
NEXT APP. DATE	PURPOSE

DATE	PHYSICIAN
TIME	CAREGIVER
RESULTS	
NEXT APP. DATE	PURPOSE

DATE	PHYSICIAN
TIME	CAREGIVER
RESULTS	
NEXT APP. DATE	PURPOSE

DATE	PHYSICIAN
TIME	CAREGIVER
RESULTS	
NEXT APP. DATE	PURPOSE

DATE	PHYSICIAN
TIME	CAREGIVER
RESULTS	
NEXT APP. DATE	PURPOSE

DATE	PHYSICIAN
TIME	CAREGIVER
RESULTS	
NEXT APP. DATE	PURPOSE

DATE	PHYSICIAN
TIME	CAREGIVER
RESULTS	
NEXT APP. DATE	PURPOSE

DATE	PHYSICIAN
TIME	CAREGIVER
RESULTS	
NEXT APP. DATE	PURPOSE

DATE	PHYSICIAN
TIME	CAREGIVER
RESULTS	
NEXT APP. DATE	PURPOSE

DATE	PHYSICIAN	
TIME	CAREGIVER	
RESULTS		
NEXT APP. DATE	PURPOSE	

DATE	PHYSICIAN	
TIME	CAREGIVER	
RESULTS		
NEXT APP. DATE	PURPOSE	

DATE	PHYSICIAN	
TIME	CAREGIVER	
RESULTS		
NEXT APP. DATE	PURPOSE	

DATE	PHYSICIAN	
TIME	CAREGIVER	
RESULTS		
NEXT APP. DATE	PURPOSE	

DATE	PHYSICIAN	
TIME	CAREGIVER	
RESULTS		
NEXT APP. DATE	PURPOSE	

DATE	PHYSICIAN
TIME	CAREGIVER
RESULTS	
NEXT APP. DATE	PURPOSE

DATE	PHYSICIAN
TIME	CAREGIVER
RESULTS	
NEXT APP. DATE	PURPOSE

DATE	PHYSICIAN
TIME	CAREGIVER
RESULTS	
NEXT APP. DATE	PURPOSE

DATE	PHYSICIAN
TIME	CAREGIVER
RESULTS	
NEXT APP. DATE	PURPOSE

DATE	PHYSICIAN
TIME	CAREGIVER
RESULTS	
NEXT APP. DATE	PURPOSE

DATE	PHYSICIAN
TIME	CAREGIVER
RESULTS	
NEXT APP. DATE	PURPOSE

DATE	PHYSICIAN
TIME	CAREGIVER
RESULTS	
NEXT APP. DATE	PURPOSE

DATE	PHYSICIAN
TIME	CAREGIVER
RESULTS	
NEXT APP. DATE	PURPOSE

DATE	PHYSICIAN
TIME	CAREGIVER
RESULTS	
NEXT APP. DATE	PURPOSE

DATE	PHYSICIAN
TIME	CAREGIVER
RESULTS	
NEXT APP. DATE	PURPOSE

DATE	PHYSICIAN
TIME	CAREGIVER
RESULTS	
NEXT APP. DATE	PURPOSE

DATE	PHYSICIAN
TIME	CAREGIVER
RESULTS	
NEXT APP. DATE	PURPOSE

DATE	PHYSICIAN
TIME	CAREGIVER
RESULTS	
NEXT APP. DATE	PURPOSE

DATE	PHYSICIAN
TIME	CAREGIVER
RESULTS	
NEXT APP. DATE	PURPOSE

DATE	PHYSICIAN
TIME	CAREGIVER
RESULTS	
NEXT APP. DATE	PURPOSE

DATE	PHYSICIAN
TIME	CAREGIVER
RESULTS	
NEXT APP. DATE	PURPOSE

DATE	PHYSICIAN
TIME	CAREGIVER
RESULTS	
NEXT APP. DATE	PURPOSE

DATE	PHYSICIAN
TIME	CAREGIVER
RESULTS	
NEXT APP. DATE	PURPOSE

DATE	PHYSICIAN
TIME	CAREGIVER
RESULTS	
NEXT APP. DATE	PURPOSE

DATE	PHYSICIAN
TIME	CAREGIVER
RESULTS	
NEXT APP. DATE	PURPOSE

DATE

PHYSICIAN

TIME

CAREGIVER

RESULTS

NEXT APP. DATE

PURPOSE

DATE

PHYSICIAN

TIME

CAREGIVER

RESULTS

NEXT APP. DATE

PURPOSE

DATE

PHYSICIAN

TIME

CAREGIVER

RESULTS

NEXT APP. DATE

PURPOSE

DATE

PHYSICIAN

TIME

CAREGIVER

RESULTS

NEXT APP. DATE

PURPOSE

DATE

PHYSICIAN

TIME

CAREGIVER

RESULTS

NEXT APP. DATE

PURPOSE

DATE	PHYSICIAN
TIMF	CAREGIVER
RESULTS	
NEXT APP. DATE	PURPOSE

DATE	PHYSICIAN
TIME	CAREGIVER
RESULTS	
NEXT APP. DATE	PURPOSE

DATE	PHYSICIAN
TIME	CAREGIVER
RESULTS	
NEXT APP. DATE	PURPOSE

DATE	PHYSICIAN
TIME	CAREGIVER
RESULTS	
NEXT APP. DATE	PURPOSE

DATE	PHYSICIAN
TIME	CAREGIVER
RESULTS	
NEXT APP. DATE	PURPOSE

DATE	PHYSICIAN
TIME	CAREGIVER
RESULTS	
NEXT APP. DATE	PURPOSE

DATE	PHYSICIAN
TIME	CAREGIVER
RESULTS	
NEXT APP. DATE	PURPOSE

DATE	PHYSICIAN
TIME	CAREGIVER
RESULTS	
NEXT APP. DATE	PURPOSE

DATE	PHYSICIAN
TIME	CAREGIVER
RESULTS	
NEXT APP. DATE	PURPOSE

DATE	PHYSICIAN
TIME	CAREGIVER
RESULTS	
NEXT APP. DATE	PURPOSE

DATE	PHYSICIAN
TIMF	CAREGIVER
RESULTS	
NEXT APP. DATE	PURPOSE

DATE	PHYSICIAN
TIME	CAREGIVER
RESULTS	
NEXT APP. DATE	PURPOSE

DATE	PHYSICIAN
TIME	CAREGIVER
RESULTS	
NEXT APP. DATE	PURPOSE

DATE	PHYSICIAN
TIME	CAREGIVER
RESULTS	
NEXT APP. DATE	PURPOSE

DATE	PHYSICIAN
TIME	CAREGIVER
RESULTS	
NEXT APP. DATE	PURPOSE

DATE	PHYSICIAN
TIME	CAREGIVER
RESULTS	
NEXT APP. DATE	PURPOSE

DATE	PHYSICIAN
TIME	CAREGIVER
RESULTS	
NEXT APP. DATE	PURPOSE

DATE	PHYSICIAN
TIME	CAREGIVER
RESULTS	
NEXT APP. DATE	PURPOSE

DATE	PHYSICIAN
TIME	CAREGIVER
RESULTS	
NEXT APP. DATE	PURPOSE

DATE	PHYSICIAN
TIME	CAREGIVER
RESULTS	
NEXT APP. DATE	PURPOSE

DATE	PHYSICIAN
TIME	CAREGIVER

RESULTS

NEXT APP. DATE	PURPOSE

DATE	PHYSICIAN
TIME	CAREGIVER

RESULTS

NEXT APP. DATE	PURPOSE

DATE	PHYSICIAN
TIME	CAREGIVER

RESULTS

NEXT APP. DATE	PURPOSE

DATE	PHYSICIAN
TIME	CAREGIVER

RESULTS

NEXT APP. DATE	PURPOSE

DATE	PHYSICIAN
TIME	CAREGIVER

RESULTS

NEXT APP. DATE	PURPOSE

DATE	PHYSICIAN
TIME	CAREGIVER
RESULTS	
NEXT APP. DATE	PURPOSE

DATE	PHYSICIAN
TIME	CAREGIVER
RESULTS	
NEXT APP. DATE	PURPOSE

DATE	PHYSICIAN
TIME	CAREGIVER
RESULTS	
NEXT APP. DATE	PURPOSE

DATE	PHYSICIAN
TIME	CAREGIVER
RESULTS	
NEXT APP. DATE	PURPOSE

DATE	PHYSICIAN
TIME	CAREGIVER
RESULTS	
NEXT APP. DATE	PURPOSE

DATE	PHYSICIAN
TIME	CAREGIVER
RESULTS	
NEXT APP. DATE	PURPOSE

DATE	PHYSICIAN
TIME	CAREGIVER
RESULTS	
NEXT APP. DATE	PURPOSE

DATE	PHYSICIAN
TIME	CAREGIVER
RESULTS	
NEXT APP. DATE	PURPOSE

DATE	PHYSICIAN
TIME	CAREGIVER
RESULTS	
NEXT APP. DATE	PURPOSE

DATE	PHYSICIAN
TIME	CAREGIVER
RESULTS	
NEXT APP. DATE	PURPOSE

DATE	PHYSICIAN
TIME	CAREGIVER
RESULTS	
NEXT APP. DATE	PURPOSE

DATE	PHYSICIAN
TIME	CAREGIVER
RESULTS	
NEXT APP. DATE	PURPOSE

DATE	PHYSICIAN
TIME	CAREGIVER
RESULTS	
NEXT APP. DATE	PURPOSE

DATE	PHYSICIAN
TIME	CAREGIVER
RESULTS	
NEXT APP. DATE	PURPOSE

DATE	PHYSICIAN
TIME	CAREGIVER
RESULTS	
NEXT APP. DATE	PURPOSE

DATE	PHYSICIAN
TIME	CAREGIVER
RESULTS	
NEXT APP. DATE	PURPOSE

DATE	PHYSICIAN
TIME	CAREGIVER
RESULTS	
NEXT APP. DATE	PURPOSE

DATE	PHYSICIAN
TIME	CAREGIVER
RESULTS	
NEXT APP. DATE	PURPOSE

DATE	PHYSICIAN
TIME	CAREGIVER
RESULTS	
NEXT APP. DATE	PURPOSE

DATE	PHYSICIAN
TIME	CAREGIVER
RESULTS	
NEXT APP. DATE	PURPOSE

Start Date

Each particular treatment is different. Some are a one-time deal, while others may be scheduled several times a week for several weeks. Knowing what day you started the treatment can also sometimes be important to have on hand in the future.

Prescribing Physician or Provider

Who is the physician that prescribed this treatment? It may seem simple at this point to track which physician prescribed which treatment, but as the treatments change and adapt, it may become harder to remember. Take a second to write it down and stay organized. Remember to put this physician's contact information in your phone book as well.

Facility

There may be instances which necessitate your need to go to a different medical facility. Chemotherapy is usually done in an infusion center. Dialysis is done at a facility specifically for dialysis. Make sure this new facility information is in your phone book.

Treatment Description

What is your treatment? Is it dialysis, radiation, or chemotherapy? How about physical therapy or lymphatic massage? Is this a one-time treatment, or will you be doing this treatment three times a week for the next eight weeks? Is it given intravenously or orally? Write down a quick, concise description of the treatment, including the type, duration, and method given if applicable.

Helpful Tip 13: Some "treatments" may also fit under the "medication" section. Example: Several chemotherapies these days are oral prescriptions that one can take regularly at home. Document this information in both the treatment and medication section.

Side Effects/Complications

This box should be filled in after the treatment. Did the patient experience nausea after the treatment? Did the patient burn, bruise, develop a rash, or have other issues? Was there constipation or diarrhea? Was the patient experiencing a lack of appetite once the treatment was complete? This is an area to document any and all side effects.

Helpful Tip 14: Write anything and everything that is unusual down in this section. You never know what is or is not a side effect (or complication) of a treatment. At your next physician or treatment appointment, bring up anything you believe to be a side effect and ask any necessary questions.

Discontinue Date (D/C)

The discontinue date, also known as the "D/C," is the date the treatment stops. If the treatment was a one-time deal, the discontinue date is the same as the starting date. If the treatment is an intravenous injection every week for the next twelve weeks, the discontinue date is the day of the last injection. For a treatment such as dialysis, which may be a regular treatment for the duration of an individual's life, there will not be a discontinue date.

START DATE	D/C	RX PHYSICIAN	FACILITY
TREATMENT			SIDE EFFECTS/COMPLICATIONS

START DATE	D/C	RX PHYSICIAN	FACILITY
TREATMENT			SIDE EFFECTS/COMPLICATIONS

START DATE	D/C	RX PHYSICIAN	FACILITY
TREATMENT			SIDE EFFECTS/COMPLICATIONS

START DATE	D/C	RX PHYSICIAN	FACILITY
TREATMENT			SIDE EFFECTS/COMPLICATIONS

START DATE	D/C	RX PHYSICIAN	FACILITY
TREATMENT			SIDE EFFECTS/COMPLICATIONS

START DATE	D/C	RX PHYSICIAN	FACILITY
TREATMENT			SIDE EFFECTS/COMPLICATIONS

START DATE	D/C	RX PHYSICIAN	FACILITY
TREATMENT			SIDE EFFECTS/COMPLICATIONS

START DATE	D/C	RX PHYSICIAN	FACILITY
TREATMENT			SIDE EFFECTS/COMPLICATIONS

START DATE	D/C	RX PHYSICIAN	FACILITY
TREATMENT		SIDE EFFECTS/COMPLICATIONS	

START DATE	D/C	RX PHYSICIAN	FACILITY
TREATMENT		SIDE EFFECTS/COMPLICATIONS	

START DATE	D/C	RX PHYSICIAN	FACILITY
TREATMENT		SIDE EFFECTS/COMPLICATIONS	

START DATE	D/C	RX PHYSICIAN	FACILITY
TREATMENT		SIDE EFFECTS/COMPLICATIONS	

START DATE	D/C	RX PHYSICIAN	FACILITY
TREATMENT		SIDE EFFECTS/COMPLICATIONS	

START DATE	D/C	RX PHYSICIAN	FACILITY
TREATMENT		SIDE EFFECTS/COMPLICATIONS	

START DATE	D/C	RX PHYSICIAN	FACILITY
TREATMENT		SIDE EFFECTS/COMPLICATIONS	

START DATE	D/C	RX PHYSICIAN	FACILITY
TREATMENT		SIDE EFFECTS/COMPLICATIONS	

START DATE	D/C	RX PHYSICIAN	FACILITY
TREATMENT		SIDE EFFECTS/COMPLICATIONS	

START DATE	D/C	RX PHYSICIAN	FACILITY
TREATMENT		SIDE EFFECTS/COMPLICATIONS	

START DATE	D/C	RX PHYSICIAN	FACILITY
TREATMENT		SIDE EFFECTS/COMPLICATIONS	

START DATE	D/C	RX PHYSICIAN	FACILITY
TREATMENT		SIDE EFFECTS/COMPLICATIONS	

START DATE	D/C	RX PHYSICIAN	FACILITY
TREATMENT		SIDE EFFECTS/COMPLICATIONS	

START DATE	D/C	RX PHYSICIAN	FACILITY
TREATMENT		SIDE EFFECTS/COMPLICATIONS	

START DATE	D/C	RX PHYSICIAN	FACILITY
TREATMENT		SIDE EFFECTS/COMPLICATIONS	

START DATE	D/C	RX PHYSICIAN	FACILITY
TREATMENT		SIDE EFFECTS/COMPLICATIONS	

START DATE	D/C	RX PHYSICIAN	FACILITY
TREATMENT		SIDE EFFECTS/COMPLICATIONS	

START DATE	D/C	RX PHYSICIAN	FACILITY
TREATMENT		SIDE EFFECTS/COMPLICATIONS	

START DATE	D/C	RX PHYSICIAN	FACILITY
TREATMENT		SIDE EFFECTS/COMPLICATIONS	

START DATE	D/C	RX PHYSICIAN	FACILITY
TREATMENT		SIDE EFFECTS/COMPLICATIONS	

START DATE	D/C	RX PHYSICIAN	FACILITY
TREATMENT		SIDE EFFECTS/COMPLICATIONS	

START DATE	D/C	RX PHYSICIAN	FACILITY
TREATMENT		SIDE EFFECTS/COMPLICATIONS	

START DATE	D/C	RX PHYSICIAN	FACILITY
TREATMENT		SIDE EFFECTS/COMPLICATIONS	

START DATE	D/C	RX PHYSICIAN	FACILITY
TREATMENT		SIDE EFFECTS/COMPLICATIONS	

START DATE	D/C	RX PHYSICIAN	FACILITY
TREATMENT		SIDE EFFECTS/COMPLICATIONS	

START DATE	D/C	RX PHYSICIAN	FACILITY
TREATMENT		SIDE EFFECTS/COMPLICATIONS	

START DATE	D/C	RX PHYSICIAN	FACILITY
TREATMENT		SIDE EFFECTS/COMPLICATIONS	

START DATE	D/C	RX PHYSICIAN	FACILITY
TREATMENT		SIDE EFFECTS/COMPLICATIONS	

START DATE	D/C	RX PHYSICIAN	FACILITY
TREATMENT		SIDE EFFECTS/COMPLICATIONS	

START DATE	D/C	RX PHYSICIAN	FACILITY
TREATMENT		SIDE EFFECTS/COMPLICATIONS	

START DATE	D/C	RX PHYSICIAN	FACILITY
TREATMENT		SIDE EFFECTS/COMPLICATIONS	

START DATE	D/C	RX PHYSICIAN	FACILITY
TREATMENT		SIDE EFFECTS/COMPLICATIONS	

START DATE	D/C	RX PHYSICIAN	FACILITY
TREATMENT		SIDE EFFECTS/COMPLICATIONS	

START DATE	D/C	RX PHYSICIAN	FACILITY
TREATMENT		SIDE EFFECTS/COMPLICATIONS	

START DATE	D/C	RX PHYSICIAN	FACILITY
TREATMENT		SIDE EFFECTS/COMPLICATIONS	

START DATE	D/C	RX PHYSICIAN	FACILITY
TREATMENT		SIDE EFFECTS/COMPLICATIONS	

START DATE	D/C	RX PHYSICIAN	FACILITY
TREATMENT		SIDE EFFECTS/COMPLICATIONS	

START DATE	D/C	RX PHYSICIAN	FACILITY
TREATMENT		SIDE EFFECTS/COMPLICATIONS	

START DATE	D/C	RX PHYSICIAN	FACILITY
TREATMENT		SIDE EFFECTS/COMPLICATIONS	

START DATE	D/C	RX PHYSICIAN	FACILITY
TREATMENT		SIDE EFFECTS/COMPLICATIONS	

START DATE	D/C	RX PHYSICIAN	FACILITY
TREATMENT			SIDE EFFECTS/COMPLICATIONS

START DATE	D/C	RX PHYSICIAN	FACILITY
TREATMENT			SIDE EFFECTS/COMPLICATIONS

START DATE	D/C	RX PHYSICIAN	FACILITY
TREATMENT			SIDE EFFECTS/COMPLICATIONS

START DATE	D/C	RX PHYSICIAN	FACILITY
TREATMENT			SIDE EFFECTS/COMPLICATIONS

START DATE	D/C	RX PHYSICIAN	FACILITY
TREATMENT			SIDE EFFECTS/COMPLICATIONS

START DATE	D/C	RX PHYSICIAN	FACILITY
TREATMENT			SIDE EFFECTS/COMPLICATIONS

START DATE	D/C	RX PHYSICIAN	FACILITY
TREATMENT			SIDE EFFECTS/COMPLICATIONS

START DATE	D/C	RX PHYSICIAN	FACILITY
TREATMENT			SIDE EFFECTS/COMPLICATIONS

START DATE	D/C	RX PHYSICIAN	FACILITY
TREATMENT		SIDE EFFECTS/COMPLICATIONS	

START DATE	D/C	RX PHYSICIAN	FACILITY
TREATMENT		SIDE EFFECTS/COMPLICATIONS	

START DATE	D/C	RX PHYSICIAN	FACILITY
TREATMENT		SIDE EFFECTS/COMPLICATIONS	

START DATE	D/C	RX PHYSICIAN	FACILITY
TREATMENT		SIDE EFFECTS/COMPLICATIONS	

START DATE	D/C	RX PHYSICIAN	FACILITY
TREATMENT		SIDE EFFECTS/COMPLICATIONS	

START DATE	D/C	RX PHYSICIAN	FACILITY
TREATMENT		SIDE EFFECTS/COMPLICATIONS	

START DATE	D/C	RX PHYSICIAN	FACILITY
TREATMENT		SIDE EFFECTS/COMPLICATIONS	

START DATE	D/C	RX PHYSICIAN	FACILITY
TREATMENT		SIDE EFFECTS/COMPLICATIONS	

START DATE	D/C	RX PHYSICIAN	FACILITY
TREATMENT			SIDE EFFECTS/COMPLICATIONS

START DATE	D/C	RX PHYSICIAN	FACILITY
TREATMENT			SIDE EFFECTS/COMPLICATIONS

START DATE	D/C	RX PHYSICIAN	FACILITY
TREATMENT			SIDE EFFECTS/COMPLICATIONS

START DATE	D/C	RX PHYSICIAN	FACILITY
TREATMENT			SIDE EFFECTS/COMPLICATIONS

START DATE	D/C	RX PHYSICIAN	FACILITY
TREATMENT			SIDE EFFECTS/COMPLICATIONS

START DATE	D/C	RX PHYSICIAN	FACILITY
TREATMENT			SIDE EFFECTS/COMPLICATIONS

START DATE	D/C	RX PHYSICIAN	FACILITY
TREATMENT			SIDE EFFECTS/COMPLICATIONS

START DATE	D/C	RX PHYSICIAN	FACILITY
TREATMENT			SIDE EFFECTS/COMPLICATIONS

START DATE	D/C	RX PHYSICIAN	FACILITY
TREATMENT			SIDE EFFECTS/COMPLICATIONS

START DATE	D/C	RX PHYSICIAN	FACILITY
TREATMENT			SIDE EFFECTS/COMPLICATIONS

START DATE	D/C	RX PHYSICIAN	FACILITY
TREATMENT			SIDE EFFECTS/COMPLICATIONS

START DATE	D/C	RX PHYSICIAN	FACILITY
TREATMENT			SIDE EFFECTS/COMPLICATIONS

START DATE	D/C	RX PHYSICIAN	FACILITY
TREATMENT			SIDE EFFECTS/COMPLICATIONS

START DATE	D/C	RX PHYSICIAN	FACILITY
TREATMENT			SIDE EFFECTS/COMPLICATIONS

START DATE	D/C	RX PHYSICIAN	FACILITY
TREATMENT			SIDE EFFECTS/COMPLICATIONS

START DATE	D/C	RX PHYSICIAN	FACILITY
TREATMENT			SIDE EFFECTS/COMPLICATIONS

Date

This may begin to sound redundant, but having a chronological order of events, written and organized, will be unbelievably helpful as you continue down this road of caregiving. Having the ability to look back and see what has occurred may help avoid complications or predicaments in the future.

Physician

This could be more than one person. It is possible that one physician prescribed a procedure and another individual conducted the procedure. If this is the case, write both names in the box. Both these individuals should be in your phone book with their specific specialties.

In the instance of a major surgery, write down the name of the surgeon. If the procedure is a biopsy, write the name of the prescribing physician and the name of the pathologist who conducted the biopsy.

Procedure

What type of procedure was conducted? The possibilities are limitless and may include, but are not limited to: biopsies, joint replacements, "-ectomies" (the act of cutting out or removing), reconstruction, or a bypass. Any exploratory or elective surgery should also be documented in this section. You never know if any of this is relevant until it has been done and time has passed. Write everything in the book so you have the information "just in case."

Chances are good that by the time you have this book in hand, several procedures have already taken place to diagnose the condition. Make sure to take a minute and add the procedures that have previously occurred.

Facility

Are you beginning to see a pattern? Always document the name of the facility in which a procedure was performed; all the facilities' contact information should be in your phonebook.

Results

What were the results or outcome of this procedure? In the case of a biopsy, were suspicious cells found? In the instance of an "-ectomy," was everything removed, or will a second procedure be required? Document any and all information the medical staff is willing to give you about the outcome of any given procedure. It is possible that no results will be available on the day of the procedure. Make a note in the appointment section (if a follow-up appointment has already been scheduled) or in the note section of this book to ask about the results of this particular procedure.

Complications

Did the procedure go as planned or were there complications during the procedure? How about after the procedure? Did the anesthesia make the individual nauseous? Were there coagulation issues? Did the individual suffer an infection or have a fever in the days following the procedure? Ask the physician if any complications occurred during the procedure and document this information for future reference. Anything out of the norm in the days preceding or following the procedure should also be documented. It never hurts to be your own advocate. Understanding the complications now may help avoid them in the future.

Follow-Up Suggestions

Usually facilities send patients home with a handout of suggestions: activities to avoid, food recommendations, and/or a timeline for recovery to name a few. Chances are good that a follow-up appointment should be made to check progress and discuss future steps.

DATE	PHYSICIAN	
PROCEDURE		FACILITY
RESULTS		
COMPLICATIONS		
FOLLOW-UP SUGGESTIONS		

DATE	PHYSICIAN	
PROCEDURE		FACILITY
RESULTS		
COMPLICATIONS		
FOLLOW-UP SUGGESTIONS		

DATE	PHYSICIAN	
PROCEDURE		FACILITY
RESULTS		
COMPLICATIONS		
FOLLOW-UP SUGGESTIONS		

DATE	PHYSICIAN	
PROCEDURE		FACILITY
RESULTS		
COMPLICATIONS		
FOLLOW-UP SUGGESTIONS		

DATE	PHYSICIAN	
PROCEDURE		FACILITY
RESULTS		
COMPLICATIONS		
FOLLOW-UP SUGGESTIONS		

DATE	PHYSICIAN	
PROCEDURE		FACILITY
RESULTS		
COMPLICATIONS		
FOLLOW-UP SUGGESTIONS		

DATE	PHYSICIAN	
PROCEDURE		FACILITY
RESULTS		
COMPLICATIONS		
FOLLOW-UP SUGGESTIONS		

DATE	PHYSICIAN	
PROCEDURE		FACILITY
RESULTS		
COMPLICATIONS		
FOLLOW-UP SUGGESTIONS		

DATE	PHYSICIAN	
PROCEDURE		FACILITY
RESULTS		
COMPLICATIONS		
FOLLOW-UP SUGGESTIONS		

DATE	PHYSICIAN	
PROCEDURE		FACILITY
RESULTS		
COMPLICATIONS		
FOLLOW-UP SUGGESTIONS		

DATE	PHYSICIAN	
PROCEDURE		FACILITY
RESULTS		
COMPLICATIONS		
FOLLOW-UP SUGGESTIONS		

DATE	PHYSICIAN	
PROCEDURE		FACILITY
RESULTS		
COMPLICATIONS		
FOLLOW-UP SUGGESTIONS		

DATE	PHYSICIAN	
PROCEDURE		FACILITY
RESULTS		
COMPLICATIONS		
FOLLOW-UP SUGGESTIONS		

DATE	PHYSICIAN	
PROCEDURE		FACILITY
RESULTS		
COMPLICATIONS		
FOLLOW-UP SUGGESTIONS		

DATE	PHYSICIAN	
PROCEDURE		FACILITY
RESULTS		
COMPLICATIONS		
FOLLOW-UP SUGGESTIONS		

DATE	PHYSICIAN	
PROCEDURE		FACILITY
RESULTS		
COMPLICATIONS		
FOLLOW-UP SUGGESTIONS		

DATE	PHYSICIAN	
PROCEDURE		FACILITY
RESULTS		
COMPLICATIONS		
FOLLOW-UP SUGGESTIONS		

DATE	PHYSICIAN	
PROCEDURE		FACILITY
RESULTS		
COMPLICATIONS		
FOLLOW-UP SUGGESTIONS		

DATE	PHYSICIAN	
PROCEDURE		FACILITY
RESULTS		
COMPLICATIONS		
FOLLOW-UP SUGGESTIONS		

DATE	PHYSICIAN	
PROCEDURE		FACILITY
RESULTS		
COMPLICATIONS		
FOLLOW-UP SUGGESTIONS		

DATE	PHYSICIAN	
PROCEDURE		FACILITY
RESULTS		
COMPLICATIONS		
FOLLOW-UP SUGGESTIONS		

DATE	PHYSICIAN	
PROCEDURE		FACILITY
RESULTS		
COMPLICATIONS		
FOLLOW-UP SUGGESTIONS		

DATE	PHYSICIAN	
PROCEDURE		FACILITY
RESULTS		
COMPLICATIONS		
FOLLOW-UP SUGGESTIONS		

DATE	PHYSICIAN	
PROCEDURE		FACILITY
RESULTS		
COMPLICATIONS		
FOLLOW-UP SUGGESTIONS		

DATE	PHYSICIAN	
PROCEDURE		FACILITY
RESULTS		
COMPLICATIONS		
FOLLOW-UP SUGGESTIONS		

DATE	PHYSICIAN
PROCEDURE	FACILITY
RESULTS	
COMPLICATIONS	
FOLLOW-UP SUGGESTIONS	

DATE	PHYSICIAN
PROCEDURE	FACILITY
RESULTS	
COMPLICATIONS	
FOLLOW-UP SUGGESTIONS	

DATE	PHYSICIAN
PROCEDURE	FACILITY
RESULTS	
COMPLICATIONS	
FOLLOW-UP SUGGESTIONS	

DATE	PHYSICIAN
PROCEDURE	FACILITY
RESULTS	
COMPLICATIONS	
FOLLOW-UP SUGGESTIONS	

DATE	PHYSICIAN
PROCEDURE	FACILITY
RESULTS	
COMPLICATIONS	
FOLLOW-UP SUGGESTIONS	

DATE	PHYSICIAN	
PROCEDURE		FACILITY
RESULTS		
COMPLICATIONS		
FOLLOW-UP SUGGESTIONS		

DATE	PHYSICIAN	
PROCEDURE		FACILITY
RESULTS		
COMPLICATIONS		
FOLLOW-UP SUGGESTIONS		

DATE	PHYSICIAN	
PROCEDURE		FACILITY
RESULTS		
COMPLICATIONS		
FOLLOW-UP SUGGESTIONS		

DATE	PHYSICIAN	
PROCEDURE		FACILITY
RESULTS		
COMPLICATIONS		
FOLLOW-UP SUGGESTIONS		

DATE	PHYSICIAN	
PROCEDURE		FACILITY
RESULTS		
COMPLICATIONS		
FOLLOW-UP SUGGESTIONS		

DATE	PHYSICIAN

PROCEDURE	FACILITY

RESULTS

COMPLICATIONS

FOLLOW-UP SUGGESTIONS

DATE	PHYSICIAN

PROCEDURE	FACILITY

RESULTS

COMPLICATIONS

FOLLOW-UP SUGGESTIONS

DATE	PHYSICIAN

PROCEDURE	FACILITY

RESULTS

COMPLICATIONS

FOLLOW-UP SUGGESTIONS

DATE	PHYSICIAN

PROCEDURE	FACILITY

RESULTS

COMPLICATIONS

FOLLOW-UP SUGGESTIONS

DATE	PHYSICIAN

PROCEDURE	FACILITY

RESULTS

COMPLICATIONS

FOLLOW-UP SUGGESTIONS

DATE	PHYSICIAN	
PROCEDURE		FACILITY
RESULTS		
COMPLICATIONS		
FOLLOW-UP SUGGESTIONS		

DATE	PHYSICIAN	
PROCEDURE		FACILITY
RESULTS		
COMPLICATIONS		
FOLLOW-UP SUGGESTIONS		

DATE	PHYSICIAN	
PROCEDURE		FACILITY
RESULTS		
COMPLICATIONS		
FOLLOW-UP SUGGESTIONS		

DATE	PHYSICIAN	
PROCEDURE		FACILITY
RESULTS		
COMPLICATIONS		
FOLLOW-UP SUGGESTIONS		

DATE	PHYSICIAN	
PROCEDURE		FACILITY
RESULTS		
COMPLICATIONS		
FOLLOW-UP SUGGESTIONS		

DATE | PHYSICIAN

PROCEDURE | FACILITY

RESULTS

COMPLICATIONS

FOLLOW-UP SUGGESTIONS

DATE | PHYSICIAN

PROCEDURE | FACILITY

RESULTS

COMPLICATIONS

FOLLOW-UP SUGGESTIONS

DATE | PHYSICIAN

PROCEDURE | FACILITY

RESULTS

COMPLICATIONS

FOLLOW-UP SUGGESTIONS

DATE | PHYSICIAN

PROCEDURE | FACILITY

RESULTS

COMPLICATIONS

FOLLOW-UP SUGGESTIONS

DATE | PHYSICIAN

PROCEDURE | FACILITY

RESULTS

COMPLICATIONS

FOLLOW-UP SUGGESTIONS

Date

What was the date you received the test or scan? This will be useful when the time comes to look back and see the progression of the disease or ailment. This date will help create a timeline and possibly help with the decision-making process in the future.

Prescribing Physician

Who was the physician that recommended the test or scans and prescribed it? This will be the individual who will give you the results.

Type

What type of test or scan did you receive? This could be anything from a complete blood panel (CBC), magnetic resonance imaging (MRI), positron emission tomography (PET), computerized axial tomography (CAT), modified barium swallow (MBS), or a simple X-ray. Make sure to note any specifics, such as whether the test was done "with contrast" or "without contrast."

Body Region

This box may not be relevant to the particular test. If not, you can disregard this box and move on. Other tests and scans are very specific to a certain region of the body, and documenting it is important to keep all records accurate. Was the scan of the brain, abdomen, pelvis, right arm, or the whole body?

If the test was something as simple as a blood test, you might want to document where they were able to find a viable blood source. Many ailing individuals become dehydrated and finding a consistent spot from which to draw blood could be helpful. It may sound simple, but as a caregiver being aware of this issue allows you to steer the phlebotomist in the correct direction.

Facility

At what facility was the scan or test performed? Make sure the contact information for this facility is in your phone book. Again, as with procedures, it is common for tests and scans to be performed in a separate facility from the prescribing physician.

Results

What were the results or outcome of the test or scan? Was there a metastasis or a definite decline in the issue? Did the blood work show the individual was deficient in something? Was the right arm broken or only sprained? Whatever the outcome, document, document, document! These results, along with the dates, will help you make appropriate decisions about care in the future. Along with the help and guidance of your physicians, you should be able to see a clearer picture of the progression of the disease.

DATE | Rx PHYSICIAN
TYPE | BODY REGION
FACILITY | RESULTS

DATE | Rx PHYSICIAN
TYPE | BODY REGION
FACILITY | RESULTS

DATE | Rx PHYSICIAN
TYPE | BODY REGION
FACILITY | RESULTS

DATE | Rx PHYSICIAN
TYPE | BODY REGION
FACILITY | RESULTS

DATE | Rx PHYSICIAN
TYPE | BODY REGION
FACILITY | RESULTS

DATE | Rx PHYSICIAN
TYPE | BODY REGION
FACILITY | RESULTS

DATE	Rx PHYSICIAN	
TYPE		BODY REGION
FACILITY		RESULTS

DATE	Rx PHYSICIAN	
TYPE		BODY REGION
FACILITY		RESULTS

DATE	Rx PHYSICIAN	
TYPE		BODY REGION
FACILITY		RESULTS

DATE	Rx PHYSICIAN	
TYPE		BODY REGION
FACILITY		RESULTS

DATE	Rx PHYSICIAN	
TYPE		BODY REGION
FACILITY		RESULTS

DATE	Rx PHYSICIAN	
TYPE		BODY REGION
FACILITY		RESULTS

DATE	Rx PHYSICIAN	
TYPE		BODY REGION
FACILITY		RESULTS

DATE	Rx PHYSICIAN	
TYPE		BODY REGION
FACILITY		RESULTS

DATE	Rx PHYSICIAN	
TYPE		BODY REGION
FACILITY		RESULTS

DATE	Rx PHYSICIAN	
TYPE		BODY REGION
FACILITY		RESULTS

DATE	Rx PHYSICIAN	
TYPE		BODY REGION
FACILITY		RESULTS

DATE	Rx PHYSICIAN	
TYPE		BODY REGION
FACILITY		RESULTS

DATE	Rx PHYSICIAN	
TYPE		BODY REGION
FACILITY		RESULTS

DATE	Rx PHYSICIAN	
TYPE		BODY REGION
FACILITY		RESULTS

DATE	Rx PHYSICIAN	
TYPE		BODY REGION
FACILITY		RESULTS

DATE	Rx PHYSICIAN	
TYPE		BODY REGION
FACILITY		RESULTS

DATE	Rx PHYSICIAN	
TYPE		BODY REGION
FACILITY		RESULTS

DATE	Rx PHYSICIAN	
TYPE		BODY REGION
FACILITY		RESULTS

DATE	Rx PHYSICIAN	
TYPE		BODY REGION
FACILITY		RESULTS

DATE	Rx PHYSICIAN	
TYPE		BODY REGION
FACILITY		RESULTS

DATE	Rx PHYSICIAN	
TYPE		BODY REGION
FACILITY		RESULTS

DATE	Rx PHYSICIAN	
TYPE		BODY REGION
FACILITY		RESULTS

DATE	Rx PHYSICIAN	
TYPE		BODY REGION
FACILITY		RESULTS

DATE	Rx PHYSICIAN	
TYPE		BODY REGION
FACILITY		RESULTS

DATE	Rx PHYSICIAN	
TYPE		BODY REGION
FACILITY		RESULTS

DATE	Rx PHYSICIAN	
TYPE		BODY REGION
FACILITY		RESULTS

DATE	Rx PHYSICIAN	
TYPE		BODY REGION
FACILITY		RESULTS

DATE	Rx PHYSICIAN	
TYPE		BODY REGION
FACILITY		RESULTS

DATE	Rx PHYSICIAN	
TYPE		BODY REGION
FACILITY		RESULTS

DATE	Rx PHYSICIAN	
TYPE		BODY REGION
FACILITY		RESULTS

DATE	Rx PHYSICIAN	
TYPE		BODY REGION
FACILITY		RESULTS

DATE	Rx PHYSICIAN	
TYPE		BODY REGION
FACILITY		RESULTS

DATE	Rx PHYSICIAN	
TYPE		BODY REGION
FACILITY		RESULTS

DATE	Rx PHYSICIAN	
TYPE		BODY REGION
FACILITY		RESULTS

DATE	Rx PHYSICIAN	
TYPE		BODY REGION
FACILITY		RESULTS

DATE	Rx PHYSICIAN	
TYPE		BODY REGION
FACILITY		RESULTS

DATE	Rx PHYSICIAN	
TYPF		BODY REGION
FACILITY		RESULTS

DATE	Rx PHYSICIAN	
TYPE		BODY REGION
FACILITY		RESULTS

DATE	Rx PHYSICIAN	
TYPE		BODY REGION
FACILITY		RESULTS

DATE	Rx PHYSICIAN	
TYPE		BODY REGION
FACILITY		RESULTS

DATE	Rx PHYSICIAN	
TYPE		BODY REGION
FACILITY		RESULTS

DATE	Rx PHYSICIAN	
TYPE		BODY REGION
FACILITY		RESULTS

DATE	Rx PHYSICIAN	
TYPE		BODY REGION
FACILITY		RESULTS

DATE	Rx PHYSICIAN	
TYPE		BODY REGION
FACILITY		RESULTS

DATE	Rx PHYSICIAN	
TYPE		BODY REGION
FACILITY		RESULTS

DATE	Rx PHYSICIAN	
TYPE		BODY REGION
FACILITY		RESULTS

DATE	Rx PHYSICIAN	
TYPE		BODY REGION
FACILITY		RESULTS

DATE	Rx PHYSICIAN	
TYPE		BODY REGION
FACILITY		RESULTS

DATE	Rx PHYSICIAN	
TYPE		BODY REGION
FACILITY		RESULTS

DATE	Rx PHYSICIAN	
TYPE		BODY REGION
FACILITY		RESULTS

DATE	Rx PHYSICIAN	
TYPE		BODY REGION
FACILITY		RESULTS

DATE	Rx PHYSICIAN	
TYPE		BODY REGION
FACILITY		RESULTS

DATE	Rx PHYSICIAN	
TYPE		BODY REGION
FACILITY		RESULTS

DATE	Rx PHYSICIAN	
TYPE		BODY REGION
FACILITY		RESULTS

DATE	Rx PHYSICIAN	
TYPE		BODY REGION
FACILITY		RESULTS

DATE	Rx PHYSICIAN	
TYPE		BODY REGION
FACILITY		RESULTS

DATE	Rx PHYSICIAN	
TYPE		BODY REGION
FACILITY		RESULTS

DATE	Rx PHYSICIAN	
TYPE		BODY REGION
FACILITY		RESULTS

DATE	Rx PHYSICIAN	
TYPE		BODY REGION
FACILITY		RESULTS

DATE	Rx PHYSICIAN	
TYPE		BODY REGION
FACILITY		RESULTS

DATE	Rx PHYSICIAN	
TYPE		BODY REGION
FACILITY		RESULTS

DATE	Rx PHYSICIAN	
TYPE		BODY REGION
FACILITY		RESULTS

DATE	Rx PHYSICIAN	
TYPE		BODY REGION
FACILITY		RESULTS

DATE	Rx PHYSICIAN	
TYPE		BODY REGION
FACILITY		RESULTS

DATE	Rx PHYSICIAN	
TYPE		BODY REGION
FACILITY		RESULTS

DATE	Rx PHYSICIAN	
TYPE		BODY REGION
FACILITY		RESULTS

Admittance and Release Date

What was the date of admission to the hospital and what was the date of release? Knowing these two dates will help you track the length of stay and the amount of time in between hospitalizations. For example: The person you are caring for begins to have severe bloating and cramping of the abdomen on a Sunday. The pain is so severe that the patient is admitted into the emergency room at a local hospital. It is discovered that the patient is retaining fluid in his/her abdominal cavity and will require a paracentesis (removal of peritoneal fluid). This simple procedure will not require hospitalization next time because you, and the doctors, are now aware of this condition. Once the procedure is done the patient is released from the hospital. The admit date and release date have been noted in the hospitalization section of this book, and the paracentesis is in the procedure section of this book.

Six weeks later, the bloat comes back. You and the patient are now informed and can go directly to your physician who can order the paracentesis, as opposed to admitting the patient to the hospital again.

Facility

To what hospital was the patient admitted? Was it your local hospital, or was it necessary to go to a specialty facility? Once the patient has been admitted, document all the pertinent information about this facility into the phone book section of this book.

Admitting Physician

Some individuals are admitted to a hospital by their personal physician, while others admit themselves through the emergency room. If you are admitted through the emergency room, ask the name of the hospitalist in charge of your case.

Symptoms

What symptoms or reasons do you have for being admitted to the hospital? In the example above, the patient was experiencing severe abdominal cramping and bloat. If the patient is in the hospital for a broken hip due to a fall, did the patient experience episodes of dizziness or nausea prior to the fall, or was it a clumsy accident? Try to document any and all relevant information.

Outcome

When being released from the hospital, the patient is usually left with after-care instructions. These instructions might include such things as changing a bandage on a daily basis, going to physical therapy two times a week for eight weeks, and seeking out a specialist to help continue a treatment process. In the example of the paracentesis above, the outcome would be: *received paracentesis due to retention of peritoneal fluid.*

ADMIT DATE	DISCHARGE DATE
ADMIT PHYSICIAN	FACILITY
SYMPTOMS	
OUTCOME	

ADMIT DATE	DISCHARGE DATE
ADMIT PHYSICIAN	FACILITY
SYMPTOMS	
OUTCOME	

ADMIT DATE	DISCHARGE DATE
ADMIT PHYSICIAN	FACILITY
SYMPTOMS	
OUTCOME	

ADMIT DATE	DISCHARGE DATE
ADMIT PHYSICIAN	FACILITY
SYMPTOMS	
OUTCOME	

ADMIT DATE	DISCHARGE DATE
ADMIT PHYSICIAN	FACILITY
SYMPTOMS	
OUTCOME	

ADMIT DATE	DISCHARGE DATE
ADMIT PHYSICIAN	FACILITY
SYMPTOMS	
OUTCOME	

ADMIT DATE	DISCHARGE DATE
ADMIT PHYSICIAN	FACILITY
SYMPTOMS	
OUTCOME	

ADMIT DATE	DISCHARGE DATE
ADMIT PHYSICIAN	FACILITY
SYMPTOMS	
OUTCOME	

ADMIT DATE	DISCHARGE DATE
ADMIT PHYSICIAN	FACILITY
SYMPTOMS	
OUTCOME	

ADMIT DATE	DISCHARGE DATE
ADMIT PHYSICIAN	FACILITY
SYMPTOMS	
OUTCOME	

ADMIT DATE	DISCHARGE DATE
ADMIT PHYSICIAN	FACILITY
SYMPTOMS	
OUTCOME	

ADMIT DATE	DISCHARGE DATE
ADMIT PHYSICIAN	FACILITY
SYMPTOMS	
OUTCOME	

ADMIT DATE | DISCHARGE DATE

ADMIT PHYSICIAN | FACILITY

SYMPTOMS

OUTCOME

ADMIT DATE | DISCHARGE DATE

ADMIT PHYSICIAN | FACILITY

SYMPTOMS

OUTCOME

ADMIT DATE | DISCHARGE DATE

ADMIT PHYSICIAN | FACILITY

SYMPTOMS

OUTCOME

ADMIT DATE | DISCHARGE DATE

ADMIT PHYSICIAN | FACILITY

SYMPTOMS

OUTCOME

ADMIT DATE | DISCHARGE DATE

ADMIT PHYSICIAN | FACILITY

SYMPTOMS

OUTCOME

ADMIT DATE | DISCHARGE DATE

ADMIT PHYSICIAN | FACILITY

SYMPTOMS

OUTCOME

ADMIT DATE | DISCHARGE DATE

ADMIT PHYSICIAN | FACILITY

SYMPTOMS

OUTCOME

ADMIT DATE | DISCHARGE DATE

ADMIT PHYSICIAN | FACILITY

SYMPTOMS

OUTCOME

ADMIT DATE | DISCHARGE DATE

ADMIT PHYSICIAN | FACILITY

SYMPTOMS

OUTCOME

ADMIT DATE | DISCHARGE DATE

ADMIT PHYSICIAN | FACILITY

SYMPTOMS

OUTCOME

ADMIT DATE | DISCHARGE DATE

ADMIT PHYSICIAN | FACILITY

SYMPTOMS

OUTCOME

ADMIT DATE | DISCHARGE DATE

ADMIT PHYSICIAN | FACILITY

SYMPTOMS

OUTCOME

ADMIT DATE	DISCHARGE DATE
ADMIT PHYSICIAN	FACILITY
SYMPTOMS	
OUTCOME	

ADMIT DATE	DISCHARGE DATE
ADMIT PHYSICIAN	FACILITY
SYMPTOMS	
OUTCOME	

ADMIT DATE	DISCHARGE DATE
ADMIT PHYSICIAN	FACILITY
SYMPTOMS	
OUTCOME	

ADMIT DATE	DISCHARGE DATE
ADMIT PHYSICIAN	FACILITY
SYMPTOMS	
OUTCOME	

ADMIT DATE	DISCHARGE DATE
ADMIT PHYSICIAN	FACILITY
SYMPTOMS	
OUTCOME	

ADMIT DATE	DISCHARGE DATE
ADMIT PHYSICIAN	FACILITY
SYMPTOMS	
OUTCOME	

ADMIT DATE	DISCHARGE DATE
ADMIT PHYSICIAN	FACILITY
SYMPTOMS	
OUTCOME	

ADMIT DATE	DISCHARGE DATE
ADMIT PHYSICIAN	FACILITY
SYMPTOMS	
OUTCOME	

ADMIT DATE	DISCHARGE DATE
ADMIT PHYSICIAN	FACILITY
SYMPTOMS	
OUTCOME	

ADMIT DATE	DISCHARGE DATE
ADMIT PHYSICIAN	FACILITY
SYMPTOMS	
OUTCOME	

ADMIT DATE	DISCHARGE DATE
ADMIT PHYSICIAN	FACILITY
SYMPTOMS	
OUTCOME	

ADMIT DATE	DISCHARGE DATE
ADMIT PHYSICIAN	FACILITY
SYMPTOMS	
OUTCOME	

Notes

Notes

Notes

Suggestions for Use

Write In Each Caregiver's "Shifts"

If there is only one caregiver for the individual, it isn't necessary to write this one person into the schedule. On the other hand, if there are several individuals involved, it can be helpful to pencil in who will be caring for the individual on what day and at what time. Let's take a look at a single week:

We know that Paulo, the husband of the patient (Cindy), will be off work every day at 5:00 PM and is available to Cindy all weekend. Her son, Austin, is available Monday and Wednesday mornings until 11:30 AM, but must be to school at noon, and he works Tuesdays, Thursdays, and Fridays. Her daughter, Amy, has made herself available to take over Monday and Wednesday at 11:30 AM to 5:00 PM, all day Tuesdays and Thursdays, but is not available until noon on Fridays. The neighbor, Mel, is available on Friday mornings for emergencies, but would prefer not to take Cindy to any appointments, unless absolutely necessary. How this should look in your day planner can be seen in (Diagram 1).

Whoever takes Cindy to her appointments will have everyone's schedule and know that scheduling a follow-up appointment on a Friday should be made for after 12:30 PM.

Month of_____ Week of_____to_____

MONDAY /	TUESDAY /	WEDNESDAY /
8.00 Austin	8.00 Amy	8.00 Austin
8.15	8.15	8.15
8.30	8.30	8.30
8.45	8.45	8.45
9.00	9.00	9.00
9.15	9.15	9.15
9.30	9.30	9.30
9.45	9.45	9.45
10.00	10.00	10.00
10.15	10.15	10.15
10.30	10.30	10.30
10.45	10.45	10.45
11.00	11.00	11.00
11.15	11.15	11.15
11.30 Amy	11.30	11.30 Amy
11.45	11.45	11.45
12.00	12.00	12.00
12.15	12.15	12.15
12.30	12.30	12.30
12.45	12.45	12.45
1.00	1.00	1.00
1.15	1.15	1.15
1.30	1.30	1.30
1.45	1.45	1.45
2.00	2.00	2.00
2.15	2.15	2.15
2.30	2.30	2.30
2.45	2.45	2.45
3.00	3.00	3.00
3.15	3.15	3.15
3.30	3.30	3.30
3.45	3.45	3.45
4.00	4.00	4.00
4.15	4.15	4.15
4.30	4.30	4.30
4.45	4.45	4.45
5.00 Paulo	5.00	5.00
5.15	5.15	5.15
5.30	5.30	5.30

Month of_____ Week of_____to_____

THURSDAY /	FRIDAY /	SATURDAY /
8.00 Amy	8.00 Mel	Paulo
8.15	8.15	
8.30	8.30	
8.45	8.45	
9.00	9.00	
9.15	9.15	
9.30	9.30	
9.45	9.45	
10.00	10.00	
10.15	10.15	
10.30	10.30	
10.45	10.45	
11.00	11.00	
11.15	11.15	
11.30	11.30	
11.45	11.45	
12.00	12.00 Amy	
12.15	12.15	
12.30	12.30	
12.45	12.45	
1.00	1.00	SUNDAY /
1.15	1.15	Paulo
1.30	1.30	
1.45	1.45	
2.00	2.00	
2.15	2.15	
2.30	2.30	
2.45	2.45	
3.00	3.00	
3.15	3.15	
3.30	3.30	
3.45	3.45	
4.00	4.00	
4.15	4.15	
4.30	4.30	
4.45	4.45	
5.00 Paulo	5.00	
5.15	5.15	
5.30	5.30	

Diagram 1. Write In Each Caregiver's "Shifts"

Write All Medical Appointments

As each day is broken into fifteen-minute increments, circle the correct time of the appointment and write in what the appointment is for and where it will be. An example of Cindy's week:

Monday, Wednesday, and Friday she needs to go to the Cancer Center for radiation at 1:45 PM. On Wednesday after her radiation, approximately 2:20 PM, she is expected at the Infusion Center for an IV treatment. Cindy must get a quick blood panel done before she is cleared for her IV treatment on Wednesdays, so it is best to go to the lab and have her blood drawn before her radiation.

Thursday there are two scans that need to occur, a bone scan at the hospital and an MRI at the imaging center. This is tricky, because Cindy must drink the contrast for the MRI in the morning (delicious orange drink), go to the nuclear department of the hospital to receive her injection of radioactive tracer, go back to the imaging center for her MRI at 10 AM, and then back to the hospital for her scan at 11:15 AM. These hectic days wear on her, but they only occur every six weeks, and she has decided she would like them done this way.

Having these appointments mapped out will help all the caregivers and the patient prepare for each day (Diagram 2).

Write All Engagements for the Individual

Chances are the patient may not be able to drive him- or herself around, but daily activities will still continue. Haircuts will still need to occur, lunch dates with friends, grocery shopping, or a weekend trip away. Having positive, fun things to do in the day planner along with the medical appointments will help everyone keep a positive outlook on the day and week ahead. Example continued:

Monday after the radiation treatment, Cindy likes to do her large grocery shopping for the week. She has a list prepared and would like to go if she is feeling up to it. If not, Amy will drop her off at home, make sure she is comfortable, and do the shopping on her own. Looking at the day planner, they notice there are no appointments or other plans on Tuesday; Cindy would really like to get her hair trimmed, but may take Tuesday off completely.

Tentatively, a Friday appointment after radiation is scheduled with Cindy's hairdresser. Because the MRI on Thursday requires fasting, Cindy is starving by the time the tests are done. Every six weeks after the scans, it is customary for Paulo, Cindy's husband, to take her to meet up with the ladies for lunch at their favorite local restaurant, where mashed potatoes are available. Mashed potatoes are her favorite!

This day planner helps you organize your day and week so the number of trips out of the house can be kept to a minimum (Diagram 3). That is, of course, only if you need to limit the number of trips. The person you are caring for may feel in relatively good health and want to continue his or her day-to-day regime just as he or she had prior to the illness. Others may not be as energetic as they once were and will require some planning to get everything accomplished.

Document Vitals

Depending upon where you find yourself in the caring process, documenting the patient's vital signs may be important. Circle the time you took the vitals and write in the results. The vital signs you may need to note are the patient's blood pressure, oxygen statistics, pulse, and temperature.

Document Unusual Behavior or Activity

If the person you are caring for experiences anything unusual, write it down. You may begin to see a pattern. Is the person forgetting very simple tasks or asking the same question several times a day? Did the individual soil the bed last night or become incontinent of bowel or bladder? Did the individual sleep twenty two hours? Was there a bloody nose? A crying spell? A laughing spell? Anything irregular should be written down and brought up to your physician. Some behavior may be irrelevant or a random event, while others may be a clue into the progression of the disease or disorder. It is not for you to decide which is random and irrelevant; write down all changes in behavior, cognition, and orientation, then consult your physician.

Include sleeping patterns. Did the patient experience a full night of restful sleep? Was it difficult to get to sleep or stay asleep? Were there

Month of_____ Week of_____to_____

MONDAY /	TUESDAY /	WEDNESDAY /
8.00 Austin	8.00 Amy	8.00 Austin
8.15	8.15	8.15
8.30	8.30	8.30
8.45	8.45	8.45
9.00	9.00	9.00
9.15	9.15	9.15
9.30	9.30	9.30
9.45	9.45	9.45
10.00	10.00	10.00
10.15	10.15	10.15
10.30	10.30	10.30
10.45	10.45	10.45
11.00	11.00	11.00
11.15	11.15	11.15
11.30 Amy	11.30	11.30 Amy
11.45	11.45	11.45
12.00	12.00	12.00
12.15	12.15	12.15
12.30	12.30	12.30
12.45	12.45	12.45
1.00	1.00	1.00
1.15	1.15	1.15 LAB - Blood Draw
1.30	1.30	1.30
1.45 Radiation	1.45	1.45 Radiation
2.00	2.00	2.00
2.15	2.15	2.15 Infusion
2.30	2.30	2.30
2.45	2.45	2.45
3.00	3.00	3.00
3.15	3.15	3.15
3.30	3.30	3.30
3.45	3.45	3.45
4.00	4.00	4.00
4.15	4.15	4.15
4.30	4.30	4.30
4.45	4.45	4.45
5.00 Paulo	5.00	5.00
5.15	5.15	5.15
5.30	5.30	5.30

Month of_____ Week of_____to_____

THURSDAY /	FRIDAY /	SATURDAY /
8.00 Amy	8.00 Mel	Paulo
(8.15) Drink Contrast	8.15	
8.30	8.30	
8.45	8.45	
9.00	9.00	
(9.15) Hospital: Tracer	9.15	
9.30	9.30	
9.45	9.45	
(10.00) Image Center: MRI	10.00	
10.15	10.15	
10.30	10.30	
10.45	10.45	
11.00	11.00	
(11.15) Hospital: Scan	11.15	
11.30	11.30	
11.45	11.45	
12.00	12.00 Amy	
12.15	12.15	
12.30	12.30	
12.45	12.45	
1.00	1.00	SUNDAY /
1.15	1.15	Paulo
1.30	1.30	
1.45	(1.45) Radiation	
2.00	2.00	
2.15	2.15	
2.30	2.30	
2.45	2.45	
3.00	3.00	
3.15	3.15	
3.30	3.30	
3.45	3.45	
4.00	4.00	
4.15	4.15	
4.30	4.30	
4.45	4.45	
5.00 Paulo	5.00	
5.15	5.15	
5.30	5.30	

Diagram 2. Write All Medical Appointments.

Month of_____ Week of_____to_____

MONDAY /	TUESDAY /	WEDNESDAY /
8.00 Austin	8.00 Amy	8.00 Austin
8.15	8.15	8.15
8.30	8.30	8.30
8.45	8.45	8.45
9.00	9.00	9.00
9.15	9.15	9.15
9.30	9.30	9.30
9.45	9.45	9.45
10.00	10.00	10.00
10.15	10.15	10.15
10.30	10.30	10.30
10.45	10.45	10.45
11.00	11.00	11.00
11.15	11.15	11.15
11.30 Amy	11.30	11.30 Amy
11.45	11.45	11.45
12.00	12.00	12.00
12.15	12.15	12.15
12.30	12.30	12.30
12.45	12.45	12.45
1.00	1.00	1.00
1.15	1.15	1.15 LAB - Blood Draw
1.30	1.30	1.30
1.45 Radiation	1.45	1.45 Radiation
2.00	2.00	2.00
2.15	2.15	2.15 Infusion
2.30 Grocery Shopping!	2.30	2.30
2.45	2.45	2.45
3.00	3.00	3.00
3.15	3.15	3.15
3.30	3.30	3.30
3.45	3.45	3.45
4.00	4.00	4.00
4.15	4.15	4.15
4.30	4.30	4.30
4.45	4.45	4.45
5.00 Paulo	5.00	5.00
5.15	5.15	5.15
5.30	5.30	5.30

Month of_____ Week of_____to_____

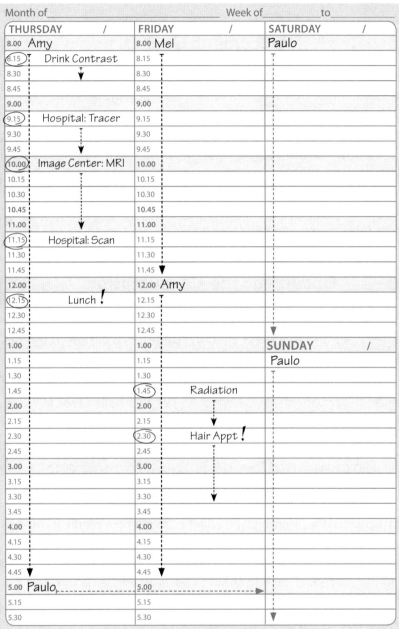

THURSDAY /	FRIDAY /	SATURDAY /
8.00 Amy	8.00 Mel	Paulo
8.15 Drink Contrast	8.15	
8.30	8.30	
8.45	8.45	
9.00	9.00	
9.15 Hospital: Tracer	9.15	
9.30	9.30	
9.45	9.45	
10.00 Image Center: MRI	10.00	
10.15	10.15	
10.30	10.30	
10.45	10.45	
11.00	11.00	
11.15 Hospital: Scan	11.15	
11.30	11.30	
11.45	11.45	
12.00	12.00 Amy	
12.15 Lunch!	12.15	
12.30	12.30	
12.45	12.45	
1.00	1.00	SUNDAY /
1.15	1.15	Paulo
1.30	1.30	
1.45	1.45 Radiation	
2.00	2.00	
2.15	2.15	
2.30	2.30 Hair Appt!	
2.45	2.45	
3.00	3.00	
3.15	3.15	
3.30	3.30	
3.45	3.45	
4.00	4.00	
4.15	4.15	
4.30	4.30	
4.45	4.45	
5.00 Paulo	5.00	
5.15	5.15	
5.30	5.30	

Diagram 3. Write All Engagements for the Individual.

nightmares, night terrors, or restless sleep? Was there sleepwalking? Was there a complaint regarding sleep, such as anxiety, pain, or fear?

Document Goals

Depending upon one's ailment, setting realistic goals and writing them in the planner may help the individual attain these goals. Individuals who have suffered a stroke may have weekly goals set by their speech therapist. Others who have had surgical procedures may have daily goals set by their physical and occupational therapist. Psychologists and family therapists may suggest projects and mood-improving exercises. Write these milestones in the day planner. Circling these goals in colored pens or adding exclamation points or stars may help improve positive thinking toward these goals; do whatever it takes!

Document the Consumption of Food and Water

Please remember that these are only suggestions of how to use this day planner. The person you are caring for may still feel vibrant, and perhaps the consumption of food is not an issue. For others, knowing when the person last ate can be a very big deal. The consumption of calories and fluids is vital to sustaining life.

Documentation of Bowel Movement and Urination

Constipation is a common side effect of many pain medications and can become a major problem if not noticed. Making a small note, like "BM" for bowel movement or "U" for urination can be helpful. Pay attention. Did the individual have to strain to have the movement, was it a "full" movement or small movement. The color of the individual's urine can give some indication of hydration. Dehydration can cause constipation, as well as dark urine with an odor. Consult your physician if you find that constipation is becoming a chronic issue. There are many remedies to treat this problem.

There are 101 ways to use the 52-week day planner. Get together with your team of caregivers and decide what information you would like in the day planner.

Other Helpful Tips

Stay Organized! Keep a copy of all medical bills, receipts, and explanations of insurance benefits. Everyone has a different system for staying organized. Some have large file cabinets; for others, staying organized just requires a shoe box full of anything that may be medically relevant. Consider investing in a small file cabinet or hanging file box. Label each hanging folder by the categories you find relevant: insurance premiums, different doctors names, pharmacies, and facilities. You may also choose to label the folders based on types of treatments, tests, scans, and medications. A sample file cabinet could look like:

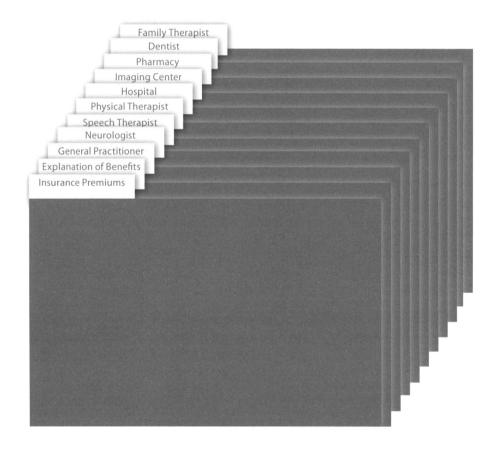

Family Therapist
Dentist
Pharmacy
Imaging Center
Hospital
Physical Therapist
Speech Therapist
Neurologist
General Practitioner
Explanation of Benefits
Insurance Premiums

If you choose to take organization to the next level, in each main file you could have folders broken into subsections:

Your level of organization is completely up to you. Knowing where to find receipts and past medical bills will be beneficial should you ever have questions regarding billing, meeting deductibles, and annual out-of-pocket expenses.

It is important to know that deductibles are met and percentages paid based on the date the provider billed the insurance company, not the date of service. This means you may believe your deductible is met when you see your chiropractor on Monday because you had an extensive operation last month that certainly had you meet your deductible. If the provider of the surgical procedure has yet to bill your insurance company at the time of your chiropractor appointment, there is a good chance that your deductible may not have been met.

The Explanation of Benefits your insurance company sends you is a synopsis of the care you have received and what has been billed. The explanation will show the date of service, type of service, amount billed by the provider, amount billed to insurance, amount the insurance paid, amount not covered by insurance, deductible you pay the provider, and/or the copayment amount. It will also show how much of your total deductible has been met to date. Do not toss these papers in the garbage because you already have the original bills filed away! If any questions arise as to why a particular invoice was billed the way it was, why a deductible wasn't quite met, or any number of other questions, the answers can usually be found in these documents.

The Most Important Tips of All:

1. **A Caregiver is only as useful to the person they are caring for as they are to themselves;** this means taking care of yourself. The role of caregiver can be very stressful, full of obstacles, and time consuming. If you do not treat your body like a temple, it will soon fall to ruin.

2. **Delegate time off:** If you find yourself being the primary caretaker with little or no time to yourself, you are setting yourself up for failure. No individual can be everywhere, for everyone, every time.

3. **Get a full night's sleep:** A full night's sleep is important for recovery. If you find yourself sleep deprived or running on empty, delegate more activities and care-related jobs to other individuals. If you find yourself in a position of caregiving during the night, be sure to get plenty of rest during the day.

4. **Have a backup team or plan:** Someone other than you should be fully aware of everything required to care for this individual. This also applies if you are the ailing individual and are caring for yourself. Either way, a time may come when you are unable to take care of one matter or another. You may require some time away, or come down with a cold; someone must be able to pick up where you left off. This

book will certainly help organize this process and help keep others abreast of what is going on in the care process. Organizing a team of caregivers to which you can delegate jobs will ensure the care process will continue smoothly should you have to be away from the situation for one reason or another.

5. **Exercise:** Simple tasks that would otherwise continue to be a part of your daily regime may be thrown to the wayside. "No time" is not an excuse to let your body go. Getting up a few minutes earlier in the morning or taking a little time in the evening to walk, jog, do yoga, swim, cross-train, or perform any other type of exercise can be very meditative and healthy. This can even be considered some "time off," an opportunity to be inside your own head and to reflect.

6. **Eat well:** Oftentimes, individuals find themselves eating fast food or processed meals because it is convenient, or not eating at all because there is "no time." Again, the "no time" excuse is not going to fly if you want to keep your mind and body healthy. Take the time to prepare fresh meals that can be eaten on the go. Many treatment facilities and hospitals have cafeterias that offer only low-quality foods. Preparing and bringing your own meals will prevent you and the ailing individual from going without a meal or being forced to consume something from a vending machine.

7. **It is okay to talk about yourself. Get a therapist:** Some believe there is a stigma attached to seeking therapy. "I don't need help" is a common excuse. You may find that the task of caregiving becomes all-encompassing in your life. Caregivers tend to put their needs to the side, projecting all of their energy toward the patient they are caring for. You may also find that the support system you once had in place is unable to comprehend the trauma you are experiencing and unable to give you the support you need. Seek the help of a professional and experience the joy of talking about yourself!

Conclusion

That was a lot of information in a short amount of time. With everything that has led you to the point of needing *The Medical Day Planner*, it is possible your head is spinning and you are a tad bit disoriented. You may be the patient requiring help keeping your personal medical journey on track, or you may be a caregiver helping a patient stay organized. Either way, do the best job you can do, stay organized, and remember to ask for help when needed. By taking these three small pieces of advice, you will make your medical voyage much more manageable.

Best of luck to you on your journey.

For more information, please visit Tory's blog at:

www.allthingscaregiver.com

Month of_____ Week of_____to_____

MONDAY /	TUESDAY /	WEDNESDAY /
8.00	8.00	8.00
8.15	8.15	8.15
8.30	8.30	8.30
8.45	8.45	8.45
9.00	9.00	9.00
9.15	9.15	9.15
9.30	9.30	9.30
9.45	9.45	9.45
10.00	10.00	10.00
10.15	10.15	10.15
10.30	10.30	10.30
10.45	10.45	10.45
11.00	11.00	11.00
11.15	11.15	11.15
11.30	11.30	11.30
11.45	11.45	11.45
12.00	12.00	12.00
12.15	12.15	12.15
12.30	12.30	12.30
12.45	12.45	12.45
1.00	1.00	1.00
1.15	1.15	1.15
1.30	1.30	1.30
1.45	1.45	1.45
2.00	2.00	2.00
2.15	2.15	2.15
2.30	2.30	2.30
2.45	2.45	2.45
3.00	3.00	3.00
3.15	3.15	3.15
3.30	3.30	3.30
3.45	3.45	3.45
4.00	4.00	4.00
4.15	4.15	4.15
4.30	4.30	4.30
4.45	4.45	4.45
5.00	5.00	5.00
5.15	5.15	5.15
5.30	5.30	5.30

52-Week Day Planner

Month of_____ Week of_____to_____

THURSDAY /	FRIDAY /	SATURDAY /
8.00	8.00	
8.15	8.15	
8.30	8.30	
8.45	8.45	
9.00	9.00	
9.15	9.15	
9.30	9.30	
9.45	9.45	
10.00	10.00	
10.15	10.15	
10.30	10.30	
10.45	10.45	
11.00	11.00	
11.15	11.15	
11.30	11.30	
11.45	11.45	
12.00	12.00	
12.15	12.15	
12.30	12.30	
12.45	12.45	
1.00	1.00	SUNDAY /
1.15	1.15	
1.30	1.30	
1.45	1.45	
2.00	2.00	
2.15	2.15	
2.30	2.30	
2.45	2.45	
3.00	3.00	
3.15	3.15	
3.30	3.30	
3.45	3.45	
4.00	4.00	
4.15	4.15	
4.30	4.30	
4.45	4.45	
5.00	5.00	
5.15	5.15	
5.30	5.30	

Month of_____ Week of_____to_____

MONDAY /	TUESDAY /	WEDNESDAY /
8.00	8.00	8.00
8.15	8.15	8.15
8.30	8.30	8.30
8.45	8.45	8.45
9.00	9.00	9.00
9.15	9.15	9.15
9.30	9.30	9.30
9.45	9.45	9.45
10.00	10.00	10.00
10.15	10.15	10.15
10.30	10.30	10.30
10.45	10.45	10.45
11.00	11.00	11.00
11.15	11.15	11.15
11.30	11.30	11.30
11.45	11.45	11.45
12.00	12.00	12.00
12.15	12.15	12.15
12.30	12.30	12.30
12.45	12.45	12.45
1.00	1.00	1.00
1.15	1.15	1.15
1.30	1.30	1.30
1.45	1.45	1.45
2.00	2.00	2.00
2.15	2.15	2.15
2.30	2.30	2.30
2.45	2.45	2.45
3.00	3.00	3.00
3.15	3.15	3.15
3.30	3.30	3.30
3.45	3.45	3.45
4.00	4.00	4.00
4.15	4.15	4.15
4.30	4.30	4.30
4.45	4.45	4.45
5.00	5.00	5.00
5.15	5.15	5.15
5.30	5.30	5.30

Month of_____ Week of_____to_____

THURSDAY /	FRIDAY /	SATURDAY /
8.00	8.00	
8.15	8.15	
8.30	8.30	
8.45	8.45	
9.00	9.00	
9.15	9.15	
9.30	9.30	
9.45	9.45	
10.00	10.00	
10.15	10.15	
10.30	10.30	
10.45	10.45	
11.00	11.00	
11.15	11.15	
11.30	11.30	
11.45	11.45	
12.00	12.00	
12.15	12.15	
12.30	12.30	
12.45	12.45	
1.00	1.00	SUNDAY /
1.15	1.15	
1.30	1.30	
1.45	1.45	
2.00	2.00	
2.15	2.15	
2.30	2.30	
2.45	2.45	
3.00	3.00	
3.15	3.15	
3.30	3.30	
3.45	3.45	
4.00	4.00	
4.15	4.15	
4.30	4.30	
4.45	4.45	
5.00	5.00	
5.15	5.15	
5.30	5.30	

Month of_____ Week of_____to_____

MONDAY /	TUESDAY /	WEDNESDAY /
8.00	8.00	8.00
8.15	8.15	8.15
8.30	8.30	8.30
8.45	8.45	8.45
9.00	9.00	9.00
9.15	9.15	9.15
9.30	9.30	9.30
9.45	9.45	9.45
10.00	10.00	10.00
10.15	10.15	10.15
10.30	10.30	10.30
10.45	10.45	10.45
11.00	11.00	11.00
11.15	11.15	11.15
11.30	11.30	11.30
11.45	11.45	11.45
12.00	12.00	12.00
12.15	12.15	12.15
12.30	12.30	12.30
12.45	12.45	12.45
1.00	1.00	1.00
1.15	1.15	1.15
1.30	1.30	1.30
1.45	1.45	1.45
2.00	2.00	2.00
2.15	2.15	2.15
2.30	2.30	2.30
2.45	2.45	2.45
3.00	3.00	3.00
3.15	3.15	3.15
3.30	3.30	3.30
3.45	3.45	3.45
4.00	4.00	4.00
4.15	4.15	4.15
4.30	4.30	4.30
4.45	4.45	4.45
5.00	5.00	5.00
5.15	5.15	5.15
5.30	5.30	5.30

Month of_____ Week of_____to_____

THURSDAY /	FRIDAY /	SATURDAY /
8.00	8.00	
8.15	8.15	
8.30	8.30	
8.45	8.45	
9.00	9.00	
9.15	9.15	
9.30	9.30	
9.45	9.45	
10.00	10.00	
10.15	10.15	
10.30	10.30	
10.45	10.45	
11.00	11.00	
11.15	11.15	
11.30	11.30	
11.45	11.45	
12.00	12.00	
12.15	12.15	
12.30	12.30	
12.45	12.45	
1.00	1.00	SUNDAY /
1.15	1.15	
1.30	1.30	
1.45	1.45	
2.00	2.00	
2.15	2.15	
2.30	2.30	
2.45	2.45	
3.00	3.00	
3.15	3.15	
3.30	3.30	
3.45	3.45	
4.00	4.00	
4.15	4.15	
4.30	4.30	
4.45	4.45	
5.00	5.00	
5.15	5.15	
5.30	5.30	

Month of_____ Week of_____to_____

MONDAY /	TUESDAY /	WEDNESDAY /
8.00	8.00	8.00
8.15	8.15	8.15
8.30	8.30	8.30
8.45	8.45	8.45
9.00	9.00	9.00
9.15	9.15	9.15
9.30	9.30	9.30
9.45	9.45	9.45
10.00	10.00	10.00
10.15	10.15	10.15
10.30	10.30	10.30
10.45	10.45	10.45
11.00	11.00	11.00
11.15	11.15	11.15
11.30	11.30	11.30
11.45	11.45	11.45
12.00	12.00	12.00
12.15	12.15	12.15
12.30	12.30	12.30
12.45	12.45	12.45
1.00	1.00	1.00
1.15	1.15	1.15
1.30	1.30	1.30
1.45	1.45	1.45
2.00	2.00	2.00
2.15	2.15	2.15
2.30	2.30	2.30
2.45	2.45	2.45
3.00	3.00	3.00
3.15	3.15	3.15
3.30	3.30	3.30
3.45	3.45	3.45
4.00	4.00	4.00
4.15	4.15	4.15
4.30	4.30	4.30
4.45	4.45	4.45
5.00	5.00	5.00
5.15	5.15	5.15
5.30	5.30	5.30

Month of_____ Week of_____to_____

THURSDAY /	FRIDAY /	SATURDAY /
8.00	8.00	
8.15	8.15	
8.30	8.30	
8.45	8.45	
9.00	9.00	
9.15	9.15	
9.30	9.30	
9.45	9.45	
10.00	10.00	
10.15	10.15	
10.30	10.30	
10.45	10.45	
11.00	11.00	
11.15	11.15	
11.30	11.30	
11.45	11.45	
12.00	12.00	
12.15	12.15	
12.30	12.30	
12.45	12.45	
1.00	1.00	SUNDAY /
1.15	1.15	
1.30	1.30	
1.45	1.45	
2.00	2.00	
2.15	2.15	
2.30	2.30	
2.45	2.45	
3.00	3.00	
3.15	3.15	
3.30	3.30	
3.45	3.45	
4.00	4.00	
4.15	4.15	
4.30	4.30	
4.45	4.45	
5.00	5.00	
5.15	5.15	
5.30	5.30	

Month of_____ Week of_____to_____

MONDAY /	TUESDAY /	WEDNESDAY /
8.00	8.00	8.00
8.15	8.15	8.15
8.30	8.30	8.30
8.45	8.45	8.45
9.00	9.00	9.00
9.15	9.15	9.15
9.30	9.30	9.30
9.45	9.45	9.45
10.00	10.00	10.00
10.15	10.15	10.15
10.30	10.30	10.30
10.45	10.45	10.45
11.00	11.00	11.00
11.15	11.15	11.15
11.30	11.30	11.30
11.45	11.45	11.45
12.00	12.00	12.00
12.15	12.15	12.15
12.30	12.30	12.30
12.45	12.45	12.45
1.00	1.00	1.00
1.15	1.15	1.15
1.30	1.30	1.30
1.45	1.45	1.45
2.00	2.00	2.00
2.15	2.15	2.15
2.30	2.30	2.30
2.45	2.45	2.45
3.00	3.00	3.00
3.15	3.15	3.15
3.30	3.30	3.30
3.45	3.45	3.45
4.00	4.00	4.00
4.15	4.15	4.15
4.30	4.30	4.30
4.45	4.45	4.45
5.00	5.00	5.00
5.15	5.15	5.15
5.30	5.30	5.30

Month of_____ Week of_____to_____

THURSDAY /	FRIDAY /	SATURDAY /
8.00	8.00	
8.15	8.15	
8.30	8.30	
8.45	8.45	
9.00	9.00	
9.15	9.15	
9.30	9.30	
9.45	9.45	
10.00	10.00	
10.15	10.15	
10.30	10.30	
10.45	10.45	
11.00	11.00	
11.15	11.15	
11.30	11.30	
11.45	11.45	
12.00	12.00	
12.15	12.15	
12.30	12.30	
12.45	12.45	
1.00	1.00	SUNDAY /
1.15	1.15	
1.30	1.30	
1.45	1.45	
2.00	2.00	
2.15	2.15	
2.30	2.30	
2.45	2.45	
3.00	3.00	
3.15	3.15	
3.30	3.30	
3.45	3.45	
4.00	4.00	
4.15	4.15	
4.30	4.30	
4.45	4.45	
5.00	5.00	
5.15	5.15	
5.30	5.30	

Month of_____ Week of_____to_____

MONDAY /	TUESDAY /	WEDNESDAY /
8.00	8.00	8.00
8.15	8.15	8.15
8.30	8.30	8.30
8.45	8.45	8.45
9.00	9.00	9.00
9.15	9.15	9.15
9.30	9.30	9.30
9.45	9.45	9.45
10.00	10.00	10.00
10.15	10.15	10.15
10.30	10.30	10.30
10.45	10.45	10.45
11.00	11.00	11.00
11.15	11.15	11.15
11.30	11.30	11.30
11.45	11.45	11.45
12.00	12.00	12.00
12.15	12.15	12.15
12.30	12.30	12.30
12.45	12.45	12.45
1.00	1.00	1.00
1.15	1.15	1.15
1.30	1.30	1.30
1.45	1.45	1.45
2.00	2.00	2.00
2.15	2.15	2.15
2.30	2.30	2.30
2.45	2.45	2.45
3.00	3.00	3.00
3.15	3.15	3.15
3.30	3.30	3.30
3.45	3.45	3.45
4.00	4.00	4.00
4.15	4.15	4.15
4.30	4.30	4.30
4.45	4.45	4.45
5.00	5.00	5.00
5.15	5.15	5.15
5.30	5.30	5.30

Month of_____ Week of_____to_____

THURSDAY /	FRIDAY /	SATURDAY /
8.00	8.00	
8.15	8.15	
8.30	8.30	
8.45	8.45	
9.00	9.00	
9.15	9.15	
9.30	9.30	
9.45	9.45	
10.00	10.00	
10.15	10.15	
10.30	10.30	
10.45	10.45	
11.00	11.00	
11.15	11.15	
11.30	11.30	
11.45	11.45	
12.00	12.00	
12.15	12.15	
12.30	12.30	
12.45	12.45	
1.00	1.00	SUNDAY /
1.15	1.15	
1.30	1.30	
1.45	1.45	
2.00	2.00	
2.15	2.15	
2.30	2.30	
2.45	2.45	
3.00	3.00	
3.15	3.15	
3.30	3.30	
3.45	3.45	
4.00	4.00	
4.15	4.15	
4.30	4.30	
4.45	4.45	
5.00	5.00	
5.15	5.15	
5.30	5.30	

Month of_____ Week of_____to_____

MONDAY /	TUESDAY /	WEDNESDAY /
8.00	8.00	8.00
8.15	8.15	8.15
8.30	8.30	8.30
8.45	8.45	8.45
9.00	9.00	9.00
9.15	9.15	9.15
9.30	9.30	9.30
9.45	9.45	9.45
10.00	10.00	10.00
10.15	10.15	10.15
10.30	10.30	10.30
10.45	10.45	10.45
11.00	11.00	11.00
11.15	11.15	11.15
11.30	11.30	11.30
11.45	11.45	11.45
12.00	12.00	12.00
12.15	12.15	12.15
12.30	12.30	12.30
12.45	12.45	12.45
1.00	1.00	1.00
1.15	1.15	1.15
1.30	1.30	1.30
1.45	1.45	1.45
2.00	2.00	2.00
2.15	2.15	2.15
2.30	2.30	2.30
2.45	2.45	2.45
3.00	3.00	3.00
3.15	3.15	3.15
3.30	3.30	3.30
3.45	3.45	3.45
4.00	4.00	4.00
4.15	4.15	4.15
4.30	4.30	4.30
4.45	4.45	4.45
5.00	5.00	5.00
5.15	5.15	5.15
5.30	5.30	5.30

Month of_____ Week of_____ to_____

THURSDAY /	FRIDAY /	SATURDAY /
8.00	8.00	
8.15	8.15	
8.30	8.30	
8.45	8.45	
9.00	9.00	
9.15	9.15	
9.30	9.30	
9.45	9.45	
10.00	10.00	
10.15	10.15	
10.30	10.30	
10.45	10.45	
11.00	11.00	
11.15	11.15	
11.30	11.30	
11.45	11.45	
12.00	12.00	
12.15	12.15	
12.30	12.30	
12.45	12.45	
1.00	1.00	SUNDAY /
1.15	1.15	
1.30	1.30	
1.45	1.45	
2.00	2.00	
2.15	2.15	
2.30	2.30	
2.45	2.45	
3.00	3.00	
3.15	3.15	
3.30	3.30	
3.45	3.45	
4.00	4.00	
4.15	4.15	
4.30	4.30	
4.45	4.45	
5.00	5.00	
5.15	5.15	
5.30	5.30	

Month of_____ Week of_____to_____

MONDAY /	TUESDAY /	WEDNESDAY /
8.00	8.00	8.00
8.15	8.15	8.15
8.30	8.30	8.30
8.45	8.45	8.45
9.00	9.00	9.00
9.15	9.15	9.15
9.30	9.30	9.30
9.45	9.45	9.45
10.00	10.00	10.00
10.15	10.15	10.15
10.30	10.30	10.30
10.45	10.45	10.45
11.00	11.00	11.00
11.15	11.15	11.15
11.30	11.30	11.30
11.45	11.45	11.45
12.00	12.00	12.00
12.15	12.15	12.15
12.30	12.30	12.30
12.45	12.45	12.45
1.00	1.00	1.00
1.15	1.15	1.15
1.30	1.30	1.30
1.45	1.45	1.45
2.00	2.00	2.00
2.15	2.15	2.15
2.30	2.30	2.30
2.45	2.45	2.45
3.00	3.00	3.00
3.15	3.15	3.15
3.30	3.30	3.30
3.45	3.45	3.45
4.00	4.00	4.00
4.15	4.15	4.15
4.30	4.30	4.30
4.45	4.45	4.45
5.00	5.00	5.00
5.15	5.15	5.15
5.30	5.30	5.30

Month of_____ Week of_____to_____

THURSDAY /	FRIDAY /	SATURDAY /
8.00	8.00	
8.15	8.15	
8.30	8.30	
8.45	8.45	
9.00	9.00	
9.15	9.15	
9.30	9.30	
9.45	9.45	
10.00	10.00	
10.15	10.15	
10.30	10.30	
10.45	10.45	
11.00	11.00	
11.15	11.15	
11.30	11.30	
11.45	11.45	
12.00	12.00	
12.15	12.15	
12.30	12.30	
12.45	12.45	
1.00	1.00	SUNDAY /
1.15	1.15	
1.30	1.30	
1.45	1.45	
2.00	2.00	
2.15	2.15	
2.30	2.30	
2.45	2.45	
3.00	3.00	
3.15	3.15	
3.30	3.30	
3.45	3.45	
4.00	4.00	
4.15	4.15	
4.30	4.30	
4.45	4.45	
5.00	5.00	
5.15	5.15	
5.30	5.30	

Month of_____ Week of_____to_____

MONDAY /	TUESDAY /	WEDNESDAY /
8.00	8.00	8.00
8.15	8.15	8.15
8.30	8.30	8.30
8.45	8.45	8.45
9.00	9.00	9.00
9.15	9.15	9.15
9.30	9.30	9.30
9.45	9.45	9.45
10.00	10.00	10.00
10.15	10.15	10.15
10.30	10.30	10.30
10.45	10.45	10.45
11.00	11.00	11.00
11.15	11.15	11.15
11.30	11.30	11.30
11.45	11.45	11.45
12.00	12.00	12.00
12.15	12.15	12.15
12.30	12.30	12.30
12.45	12.45	12.45
1.00	1.00	1.00
1.15	1.15	1.15
1.30	1.30	1.30
1.45	1.45	1.45
2.00	2.00	2.00
2.15	2.15	2.15
2.30	2.30	2.30
2.45	2.45	2.45
3.00	3.00	3.00
3.15	3.15	3.15
3.30	3.30	3.30
3.45	3.45	3.45
4.00	4.00	4.00
4.15	4.15	4.15
4.30	4.30	4.30
4.45	4.45	4.45
5.00	5.00	5.00
5.15	5.15	5.15
5.30	5.30	5.30

Month of_____ Week of_____to_____

THURSDAY /	FRIDAY /	SATURDAY /
8.00	8.00	
8.15	8.15	
8.30	8.30	
8.45	8.45	
9.00	9.00	
9.15	9.15	
9.30	9.30	
9.45	9.45	
10.00	10.00	
10.15	10.15	
10.30	10.30	
10.45	10.45	
11.00	11.00	
11.15	11.15	
11.30	11.30	
11.45	11.45	
12.00	12.00	
12.15	12.15	
12.30	12.30	
12.45	12.45	
1.00	1.00	SUNDAY /
1.15	1.15	
1.30	1.30	
1.45	1.45	
2.00	2.00	
2.15	2.15	
2.30	2.30	
2.45	2.45	
3.00	3.00	
3.15	3.15	
3.30	3.30	
3.45	3.45	
4.00	4.00	
4.15	4.15	
4.30	4.30	
4.45	4.45	
5.00	5.00	
5.15	5.15	
5.30	5.30	

Month of_____ Week of_____to_____

MONDAY /	TUESDAY /	WEDNESDAY /
8.00	8.00	8.00
8.15	8.15	8.15
8.30	8.30	8.30
8.45	8.45	8.45
9.00	9.00	9.00
9.15	9.15	9.15
9.30	9.30	9.30
9.45	9.45	9.45
10.00	10.00	10.00
10.15	10.15	10.15
10.30	10.30	10.30
10.45	10.45	10.45
11.00	11.00	11.00
11.15	11.15	11.15
11.30	11.30	11.30
11.45	11.45	11.45
12.00	12.00	12.00
12.15	12.15	12.15
12.30	12.30	12.30
12.45	12.45	12.45
1.00	1.00	1.00
1.15	1.15	1.15
1.30	1.30	1.30
1.45	1.45	1.45
2.00	2.00	2.00
2.15	2.15	2.15
2.30	2.30	2.30
2.45	2.45	2.45
3.00	3.00	3.00
3.15	3.15	3.15
3.30	3.30	3.30
3.45	3.45	3.45
4.00	4.00	4.00
4.15	4.15	4.15
4.30	4.30	4.30
4.45	4.45	4.45
5.00	5.00	5.00
5.15	5.15	5.15
5.30	5.30	5.30

Month of_____ Week of_____to_____

THURSDAY /	FRIDAY /	SATURDAY /
8.00	8.00	
8.15	8.15	
8.30	8.30	
8.45	8.45	
9.00	9.00	
9.15	9.15	
9.30	9.30	
9.45	9.45	
10.00	10.00	
10.15	10.15	
10.30	10.30	
10.45	10.45	
11.00	11.00	
11.15	11.15	
11.30	11.30	
11.45	11.45	
12.00	12.00	
12.15	12.15	
12.30	12.30	
12.45	12.45	
1.00	1.00	SUNDAY /
1.15	1.15	
1.30	1.30	
1.45	1.45	
2.00	2.00	
2.15	2.15	
2.30	2.30	
2.45	2.45	
3.00	3.00	
3.15	3.15	
3.30	3.30	
3.45	3.45	
4.00	4.00	
4.15	4.15	
4.30	4.30	
4.45	4.45	
5.00	5.00	
5.15	5.15	
5.30	5.30	

Month of_____ Week of_____to_____

MONDAY /	TUESDAY /	WEDNESDAY /
8.00	8.00	8.00
8.15	8.15	8.15
8.30	8.30	8.30
8.45	8.45	8.45
9.00	9.00	9.00
9.15	9.15	9.15
9.30	9.30	9.30
9.45	9.45	9.45
10.00	10.00	10.00
10.15	10.15	10.15
10.30	10.30	10.30
10.45	10.45	10.45
11.00	11.00	11.00
11.15	11.15	11.15
11.30	11.30	11.30
11.45	11.45	11.45
12.00	12.00	12.00
12.15	12.15	12.15
12.30	12.30	12.30
12.45	12.45	12.45
1.00	1.00	1.00
1.15	1.15	1.15
1.30	1.30	1.30
1.45	1.45	1.45
2.00	2.00	2.00
2.15	2.15	2.15
2.30	2.30	2.30
2.45	2.45	2.45
3.00	3.00	3.00
3.15	3.15	3.15
3.30	3.30	3.30
3.45	3.45	3.45
4.00	4.00	4.00
4.15	4.15	4.15
4.30	4.30	4.30
4.45	4.45	4.45
5.00	5.00	5.00
5.15	5.15	5.15
5.30	5.30	5.30

Month of_____ Week of_____to_____

THURSDAY /	FRIDAY /	SATURDAY /
8.00	8.00	
8.15	8.15	
8.30	8.30	
8.45	8.45	
9.00	9.00	
9.15	9.15	
9.30	9.30	
9.45	9.45	
10.00	10.00	
10.15	10.15	
10.30	10.30	
10.45	10.45	
11.00	11.00	
11.15	11.15	
11.30	11.30	
11.45	11.45	
12.00	12.00	
12.15	12.15	
12.30	12.30	
12.45	12.45	
1.00	1.00	SUNDAY /
1.15	1.15	
1.30	1.30	
1.45	1.45	
2.00	2.00	
2.15	2.15	
2.30	2.30	
2.45	2.45	
3.00	3.00	
3.15	3.15	
3.30	3.30	
3.45	3.45	
4.00	4.00	
4.15	4.15	
4.30	4.30	
4.45	4.45	
5.00	5.00	
5.15	5.15	
5.30	5.30	

Month of_____ Week of_____to_____

MONDAY /	TUESDAY /	WEDNESDAY /
8.00	8.00	8.00
8.15	8.15	8.15
8.30	8.30	8.30
8.45	8.45	8.45
9.00	9.00	9.00
9.15	9.15	9.15
9.30	9.30	9.30
9.45	9.45	9.45
10.00	10.00	10.00
10.15	10.15	10.15
10.30	10.30	10.30
10.45	10.45	10.45
11.00	11.00	11.00
11.15	11.15	11.15
11.30	11.30	11.30
11.45	11.45	11.45
12.00	12.00	12.00
12.15	12.15	12.15
12.30	12.30	12.30
12.45	12.45	12.45
1.00	1.00	1.00
1.15	1.15	1.15
1.30	1.30	1.30
1.45	1.45	1.45
2.00	2.00	2.00
2.15	2.15	2.15
2.30	2.30	2.30
2.45	2.45	2.45
3.00	3.00	3.00
3.15	3.15	3.15
3.30	3.30	3.30
3.45	3.45	3.45
4.00	4.00	4.00
4.15	4.15	4.15
4.30	4.30	4.30
4.45	4.45	4.45
5.00	5.00	5.00
5.15	5.15	5.15
5.30	5.30	5.30

Month of_____ Week of_____to_____

THURSDAY /	FRIDAY /	SATURDAY /
8.00	8.00	
8.15	8.15	
8.30	8.30	
8.45	8.45	
9.00	9.00	
9.15	9.15	
9.30	9.30	
9.45	9.45	
10.00	10.00	
10.15	10.15	
10.30	10.30	
10.45	10.45	
11.00	11.00	
11.15	11.15	
11.30	11.30	
11.45	11.45	
12.00	12.00	
12.15	12.15	
12.30	12.30	
12.45	12.45	
1.00	1.00	SUNDAY /
1.15	1.15	
1.30	1.30	
1.45	1.45	
2.00	2.00	
2.15	2.15	
2.30	2.30	
2.45	2.45	
3.00	3.00	
3.15	3.15	
3.30	3.30	
3.45	3.45	
4.00	4.00	
4.15	4.15	
4.30	4.30	
4.45	4.45	
5.00	5.00	
5.15	5.15	
5.30	5.30	

52-Week Day Planner

Month of_____ Week of_____to_____

MONDAY /	TUESDAY /	WEDNESDAY /
8.00	8.00	8.00
8.15	8.15	8.15
8.30	8.30	8.30
8.45	8.45	8.45
9.00	9.00	9.00
9.15	9.15	9.15
9.30	9.30	9.30
9.45	9.45	9.45
10.00	10.00	10.00
10.15	10.15	10.15
10.30	10.30	10.30
10.45	10.45	10.45
11.00	11.00	11.00
11.15	11.15	11.15
11.30	11.30	11.30
11.45	11.45	11.45
12.00	12.00	12.00
12.15	12.15	12.15
12.30	12.30	12.30
12.45	12.45	12.45
1.00	1.00	1.00
1.15	1.15	1.15
1.30	1.30	1.30
1.45	1.45	1.45
2.00	2.00	2.00
2.15	2.15	2.15
2.30	2.30	2.30
2.45	2.45	2.45
3.00	3.00	3.00
3.15	3.15	3.15
3.30	3.30	3.30
3.45	3.45	3.45
4.00	4.00	4.00
4.15	4.15	4.15
4.30	4.30	4.30
4.45	4.45	4.45
5.00	5.00	5.00
5.15	5.15	5.15
5.30	5.30	5.30

Month of_____ Week of_____to_____

THURSDAY /	FRIDAY /	SATURDAY /
8.00	8.00	
8.15	8.15	
8.30	8.30	
8.45	8.45	
9.00	9.00	
9.15	9.15	
9.30	9.30	
9.45	9.45	
10.00	10.00	
10.15	10.15	
10.30	10.30	
10.45	10.45	
11.00	11.00	
11.15	11.15	
11.30	11.30	
11.45	11.45	
12.00	12.00	
12.15	12.15	
12.30	12.30	
12.45	12.45	
1.00	1.00	SUNDAY /
1.15	1.15	
1.30	1.30	
1.45	1.45	
2.00	2.00	
2.15	2.15	
2.30	2.30	
2.45	2.45	
3.00	3.00	
3.15	3.15	
3.30	3.30	
3.45	3.45	
4.00	4.00	
4.15	4.15	
4.30	4.30	
4.45	4.45	
5.00	5.00	
5.15	5.15	
5.30	5.30	

Month of_____ Week of_____to_____

MONDAY /	TUESDAY /	WEDNESDAY /
8.00	8.00	8.00
8.15	8.15	8.15
8.30	8.30	8.30
8.45	8.45	8.45
9.00	9.00	9.00
9.15	9.15	9.15
9.30	9.30	9.30
9.45	9.45	9.45
10.00	10.00	10.00
10.15	10.15	10.15
10.30	10.30	10.30
10.45	10.45	10.45
11.00	11.00	11.00
11.15	11.15	11.15
11.30	11.30	11.30
11.45	11.45	11.45
12.00	12.00	12.00
12.15	12.15	12.15
12.30	12.30	12.30
12.45	12.45	12.45
1.00	1.00	1.00
1.15	1.15	1.15
1.30	1.30	1.30
1.45	1.45	1.45
2.00	2.00	2.00
2.15	2.15	2.15
2.30	2.30	2.30
2.45	2.45	2.45
3.00	3.00	3.00
3.15	3.15	3.15
3.30	3.30	3.30
3.45	3.45	3.45
4.00	4.00	4.00
4.15	4.15	4.15
4.30	4.30	4.30
4.45	4.45	4.45
5.00	5.00	5.00
5.15	5.15	5.15
5.30	5.30	5.30

Month of_____ Week of_____to_____

THURSDAY /	FRIDAY /	SATURDAY /
8.00	8.00	
8.15	8.15	
8.30	8.30	
8.45	8.45	
9.00	9.00	
9.15	9.15	
9.30	9.30	
9.45	9.45	
10.00	10.00	
10.15	10.15	
10.30	10.30	
10.45	10.45	
11.00	11.00	
11.15	11.15	
11.30	11.30	
11.45	11.45	
12.00	12.00	
12.15	12.15	
12.30	12.30	
12.45	12.45	
1.00	1.00	SUNDAY /
1.15	1.15	
1.30	1.30	
1.45	1.45	
2.00	2.00	
2.15	2.15	
2.30	2.30	
2.45	2.45	
3.00	3.00	
3.15	3.15	
3.30	3.30	
3.45	3.45	
4.00	4.00	
4.15	4.15	
4.30	4.30	
4.45	4.45	
5.00	5.00	
5.15	5.15	
5.30	5.30	

Month of_____ Week of_____to_____

MONDAY /	TUESDAY /	WEDNESDAY /
8.00	8.00	8.00
8.15	8.15	8.15
8.30	8.30	8.30
8.45	8.45	8.45
9.00	9.00	9.00
9.15	9.15	9.15
9.30	9.30	9.30
9.45	9.45	9.45
10.00	10.00	10.00
10.15	10.15	10.15
10.30	10.30	10.30
10.45	10.45	10.45
11.00	11.00	11.00
11.15	11.15	11.15
11.30	11.30	11.30
11.45	11.45	11.45
12.00	12.00	12.00
12.15	12.15	12.15
12.30	12.30	12.30
12.45	12.45	12.45
1.00	1.00	1.00
1.15	1.15	1.15
1.30	1.30	1.30
1.45	1.45	1.45
2.00	2.00	2.00
2.15	2.15	2.15
2.30	2.30	2.30
2.45	2.45	2.45
3.00	3.00	3.00
3.15	3.15	3.15
3.30	3.30	3.30
3.45	3.45	3.45
4.00	4.00	4.00
4.15	4.15	4.15
4.30	4.30	4.30
4.45	4.45	4.45
5.00	5.00	5.00
5.15	5.15	5.15
5.30	5.30	5.30

Month of_____ Week of_____to_____

THURSDAY /	FRIDAY /	SATURDAY /
8.00	8.00	
8.15	8.15	
8.30	8.30	
8.45	8.45	
9.00	9.00	
9.15	9.15	
9.30	9.30	
9.45	9.45	
10.00	10.00	
10.15	10.15	
10.30	10.30	
10.45	10.45	
11.00	11.00	
11.15	11.15	
11.30	11.30	
11.45	11.45	
12.00	12.00	
12.15	12.15	
12.30	12.30	
12.45	12.45	
1.00	1.00	SUNDAY /
1.15	1.15	
1.30	1.30	
1.45	1.45	
2.00	2.00	
2.15	2.15	
2.30	2.30	
2.45	2.45	
3.00	3.00	
3.15	3.15	
3.30	3.30	
3.45	3.45	
4.00	4.00	
4.15	4.15	
4.30	4.30	
4.45	4.45	
5.00	5.00	
5.15	5.15	
5.30	5.30	

Month of_____ Week of_____to_____

MONDAY /	TUESDAY /	WEDNESDAY /
8.00	8.00	8.00
8.15	8.15	8.15
8.30	8.30	8.30
8.45	8.45	8.45
9.00	9.00	9.00
9.15	9.15	9.15
9.30	9.30	9.30
9.45	9.45	9.45
10.00	10.00	10.00
10.15	10.15	10.15
10.30	10.30	10.30
10.45	10.45	10.45
11.00	11.00	11.00
11.15	11.15	11.15
11.30	11.30	11.30
11.45	11.45	11.45
12.00	12.00	12.00
12.15	12.15	12.15
12.30	12.30	12.30
12.45	12.45	12.45
1.00	1.00	1.00
1.15	1.15	1.15
1.30	1.30	1.30
1.45	1.45	1.45
2.00	2.00	2.00
2.15	2.15	2.15
2.30	2.30	2.30
2.45	2.45	2.45
3.00	3.00	3.00
3.15	3.15	3.15
3.30	3.30	3.30
3.45	3.45	3.45
4.00	4.00	4.00
4.15	4.15	4.15
4.30	4.30	4.30
4.45	4.45	4.45
5.00	5.00	5.00
5.15	5.15	5.15
5.30	5.30	5.30

Month of_____ Week of_____to_____

THURSDAY /	FRIDAY /	SATURDAY /
8.00	8.00	
8.15	8.15	
8.30	8.30	
8.45	8.45	
9.00	9.00	
9.15	9.15	
9.30	9.30	
9.45	9.45	
10.00	10.00	
10.15	10.15	
10.30	10.30	
10.45	10.45	
11.00	11.00	
11.15	11.15	
11.30	11.30	
11.45	11.45	
12.00	12.00	
12.15	12.15	
12.30	12.30	
12.45	12.45	
1.00	1.00	SUNDAY /
1.15	1.15	
1.30	1.30	
1.45	1.45	
2.00	2.00	
2.15	2.15	
2.30	2.30	
2.45	2.45	
3.00	3.00	
3.15	3.15	
3.30	3.30	
3.45	3.45	
4.00	4.00	
4.15	4.15	
4.30	4.30	
4.45	4.45	
5.00	5.00	
5.15	5.15	
5.30	5.30	

Month of_____ Week of_____to_____

MONDAY /	TUESDAY /	WEDNESDAY /
8.00	8.00	8.00
8.15	8.15	8.15
8.30	8.30	8.30
8.45	8.45	8.45
9.00	9.00	9.00
9.15	9.15	9.15
9.30	9.30	9.30
9.45	9.45	9.45
10.00	10.00	10.00
10.15	10.15	10.15
10.30	10.30	10.30
10.45	10.45	10.45
11.00	11.00	11.00
11.15	11.15	11.15
11.30	11.30	11.30
11.45	11.45	11.45
12.00	12.00	12.00
12.15	12.15	12.15
12.30	12.30	12.30
12.45	12.45	12.45
1.00	1.00	1.00
1.15	1.15	1.15
1.30	1.30	1.30
1.45	1.45	1.45
2.00	2.00	2.00
2.15	2.15	2.15
2.30	2.30	2.30
2.45	2.45	2.45
3.00	3.00	3.00
3.15	3.15	3.15
3.30	3.30	3.30
3.45	3.45	3.45
4.00	4.00	4.00
4.15	4.15	4.15
4.30	4.30	4.30
4.45	4.45	4.45
5.00	5.00	5.00
5.15	5.15	5.15
5.30	5.30	5.30

Month of_____ Week of_____to_____

THURSDAY /	FRIDAY /	SATURDAY /
8.00	8.00	
8.15	8.15	
8.30	8.30	
8.45	8.45	
9.00	9.00	
9.15	9.15	
9.30	9.30	
9.45	9.45	
10.00	10.00	
10.15	10.15	
10.30	10.30	
10.45	10.45	
11.00	11.00	
11.15	11.15	
11.30	11.30	
11.45	11.45	
12.00	12.00	
12.15	12.15	
12.30	12.30	
12.45	12.45	
1.00	1.00	SUNDAY /
1.15	1.15	
1.30	1.30	
1.45	1.45	
2.00	2.00	
2.15	2.15	
2.30	2.30	
2.45	2.45	
3.00	3.00	
3.15	3.15	
3.30	3.30	
3.45	3.45	
4.00	4.00	
4.15	4.15	
4.30	4.30	
4.45	4.45	
5.00	5.00	
5.15	5.15	
5.30	5.30	

Month of_____ Week of_____to_____

MONDAY /	TUESDAY /	WEDNESDAY /
8.00	8.00	8.00
8.15	8.15	8.15
8.30	8.30	8.30
8.45	8.45	8.45
9.00	9.00	9.00
9.15	9.15	9.15
9.30	9.30	9.30
9.45	9.45	9.45
10.00	10.00	10.00
10.15	10.15	10.15
10.30	10.30	10.30
10.45	10.45	10.45
11.00	11.00	11.00
11.15	11.15	11.15
11.30	11.30	11.30
11.45	11.45	11.45
12.00	12.00	12.00
12.15	12.15	12.15
12.30	12.30	12.30
12.45	12.45	12.45
1.00	1.00	1.00
1.15	1.15	1.15
1.30	1.30	1.30
1.45	1.45	1.45
2.00	2.00	2.00
2.15	2.15	2.15
2.30	2.30	2.30
2.45	2.45	2.45
3.00	3.00	3.00
3.15	3.15	3.15
3.30	3.30	3.30
3.45	3.45	3.45
4.00	4.00	4.00
4.15	4.15	4.15
4.30	4.30	4.30
4.45	4.45	4.45
5.00	5.00	5.00
5.15	5.15	5.15
5.30	5.30	5.30

Month of_____ Week of_____to_____

THURSDAY /	FRIDAY /	SATURDAY /
8.00	8.00	
8.15	8.15	
8.30	8.30	
8.45	8.45	
9.00	9.00	
9.15	9.15	
9.30	9.30	
9.45	9.45	
10.00	10.00	
10.15	10.15	
10.30	10.30	
10.45	10.45	
11.00	11.00	
11.15	11.15	
11.30	11.30	
11.45	11.45	
12.00	12.00	
12.15	12.15	
12.30	12.30	
12.45	12.45	
1.00	1.00	SUNDAY /
1.15	1.15	
1.30	1.30	
1.45	1.45	
2.00	2.00	
2.15	2.15	
2.30	2.30	
2.45	2.45	
3.00	3.00	
3.15	3.15	
3.30	3.30	
3.45	3.45	
4.00	4.00	
4.15	4.15	
4.30	4.30	
4.45	4.45	
5.00	5.00	
5.15	5.15	
5.30	5.30	

Month of_____ Week of_____to_____

MONDAY /	TUESDAY /	WEDNESDAY /
8.00	8.00	8.00
8.15	8.15	8.15
8.30	8.30	8.30
8.45	8.45	8.45
9.00	9.00	9.00
9.15	9.15	9.15
9.30	9.30	9.30
9.45	9.45	9.45
10.00	10.00	10.00
10.15	10.15	10.15
10.30	10.30	10.30
10.45	10.45	10.45
11.00	11.00	11.00
11.15	11.15	11.15
11.30	11.30	11.30
11.45	11.45	11.45
12.00	12.00	12.00
12.15	12.15	12.15
12.30	12.30	12.30
12.45	12.45	12.45
1.00	1.00	1.00
1.15	1.15	1.15
1.30	1.30	1.30
1.45	1.45	1.45
2.00	2.00	2.00
2.15	2.15	2.15
2.30	2.30	2.30
2.45	2.45	2.45
3.00	3.00	3.00
3.15	3.15	3.15
3.30	3.30	3.30
3.45	3.45	3.45
4.00	4.00	4.00
4.15	4.15	4.15
4.30	4.30	4.30
4.45	4.45	4.45
5.00	5.00	5.00
5.15	5.15	5.15
5.30	5.30	5.30

Month of_____ Week of_____to_____

THURSDAY /	FRIDAY /	SATURDAY /
8.00	8.00	
8.15	8.15	
8.30	8.30	
8.45	8.45	
9.00	9.00	
9.15	9.15	
9.30	9.30	
9.45	9.45	
10.00	10.00	
10.15	10.15	
10.30	10.30	
10.45	10.45	
11.00	11.00	
11.15	11.15	
11.30	11.30	
11.45	11.45	
12.00	12.00	
12.15	12.15	
12.30	12.30	
12.45	12.45	
1.00	1.00	SUNDAY /
1.15	1.15	
1.30	1.30	
1.45	1.45	
2.00	2.00	
2.15	2.15	
2.30	2.30	
2.45	2.45	
3.00	3.00	
3.15	3.15	
3.30	3.30	
3.45	3.45	
4.00	4.00	
4.15	4.15	
4.30	4.30	
4.45	4.45	
5.00	5.00	
5.15	5.15	
5.30	5.30	

Month of_____ Week of_____to_____

MONDAY /	TUESDAY /	WEDNESDAY /
8.00	8.00	8.00
8.15	8.15	8.15
8.30	8.30	8.30
8.45	8.45	8.45
9.00	9.00	9.00
9.15	9.15	9.15
9.30	9.30	9.30
9.45	9.45	9.45
10.00	10.00	10.00
10.15	10.15	10.15
10.30	10.30	10.30
10.45	10.45	10.45
11.00	11.00	11.00
11.15	11.15	11.15
11.30	11.30	11.30
11.45	11.45	11.45
12.00	12.00	12.00
12.15	12.15	12.15
12.30	12.30	12.30
12.45	12.45	12.45
1.00	1.00	1.00
1.15	1.15	1.15
1.30	1.30	1.30
1.45	1.45	1.45
2.00	2.00	2.00
2.15	2.15	2.15
2.30	2.30	2.30
2.45	2.45	2.45
3.00	3.00	3.00
3.15	3.15	3.15
3.30	3.30	3.30
3.45	3.45	3.45
4.00	4.00	4.00
4.15	4.15	4.15
4.30	4.30	4.30
4.45	4.45	4.45
5.00	5.00	5.00
5.15	5.15	5.15
5.30	5.30	5.30

Month of_____ Week of_____to_____

THURSDAY /	FRIDAY /	SATURDAY /
8.00	8.00	
8.15	8.15	
8.30	8.30	
8.45	8.45	
9.00	9.00	
9.15	9.15	
9.30	9.30	
9.45	9.45	
10.00	10.00	
10.15	10.15	
10.30	10.30	
10.45	10.45	
11.00	11.00	
11.15	11.15	
11.30	11.30	
11.45	11.45	
12.00	12.00	
12.15	12.15	
12.30	12.30	
12.45	12.45	
1.00	1.00	SUNDAY /
1.15	1.15	
1.30	1.30	
1.45	1.45	
2.00	2.00	
2.15	2.15	
2.30	2.30	
2.45	2.45	
3.00	3.00	
3.15	3.15	
3.30	3.30	
3.45	3.45	
4.00	4.00	
4.15	4.15	
4.30	4.30	
4.45	4.45	
5.00	5.00	
5.15	5.15	
5.30	5.30	

Month of_____ Week of_____to_____

MONDAY /	TUESDAY /	WEDNESDAY /
8.00	8.00	8.00
8.15	8.15	8.15
8.30	8.30	8.30
8.45	8.45	8.45
9.00	9.00	9.00
9.15	9.15	9.15
9.30	9.30	9.30
9.45	9.45	9.45
10.00	10.00	10.00
10.15	10.15	10.15
10.30	10.30	10.30
10.45	10.45	10.45
11.00	11.00	11.00
11.15	11.15	11.15
11.30	11.30	11.30
11.45	11.45	11.45
12.00	12.00	12.00
12.15	12.15	12.15
12.30	12.30	12.30
12.45	12.45	12.45
1.00	1.00	1.00
1.15	1.15	1.15
1.30	1.30	1.30
1.45	1.45	1.45
2.00	2.00	2.00
2.15	2.15	2.15
2.30	2.30	2.30
2.45	2.45	2.45
3.00	3.00	3.00
3.15	3.15	3.15
3.30	3.30	3.30
3.45	3.45	3.45
4.00	4.00	4.00
4.15	4.15	4.15
4.30	4.30	4.30
4.45	4.45	4.45
5.00	5.00	5.00
5.15	5.15	5.15
5.30	5.30	5.30

Month of_____ Week of_____to_____

THURSDAY /	FRIDAY /	SATURDAY /
8.00	8.00	
8.15	8.15	
8.30	8.30	
8.45	8.45	
9.00	9.00	
9.15	9.15	
9.30	9.30	
9.45	9.45	
10.00	10.00	
10.15	10.15	
10.30	10.30	
10.45	10.45	
11.00	11.00	
11.15	11.15	
11.30	11.30	
11.45	11.45	
12.00	12.00	
12.15	12.15	
12.30	12.30	
12.45	12.45	
1.00	1.00	SUNDAY /
1.15	1.15	
1.30	1.30	
1.45	1.45	
2.00	2.00	
2.15	2.15	
2.30	2.30	
2.45	2.45	
3.00	3.00	
3.15	3.15	
3.30	3.30	
3.45	3.45	
4.00	4.00	
4.15	4.15	
4.30	4.30	
4.45	4.45	
5.00	5.00	
5.15	5.15	
5.30	5.30	

Month of_____ Week of_____to_____

MONDAY /	TUESDAY /	WEDNESDAY /
8.00	8.00	8.00
8.15	8.15	8.15
8.30	8.30	8.30
8.45	8.45	8.45
9.00	9.00	9.00
9.15	9.15	9.15
9.30	9.30	9.30
9.45	9.45	9.45
10.00	10.00	10.00
10.15	10.15	10.15
10.30	10.30	10.30
10.45	10.45	10.45
11.00	11.00	11.00
11.15	11.15	11.15
11.30	11.30	11.30
11.45	11.45	11.45
12.00	12.00	12.00
12.15	12.15	12.15
12.30	12.30	12.30
12.45	12.45	12.45
1.00	1.00	1.00
1.15	1.15	1.15
1.30	1.30	1.30
1.45	1.45	1.45
2.00	2.00	2.00
2.15	2.15	2.15
2.30	2.30	2.30
2.45	2.45	2.45
3.00	3.00	3.00
3.15	3.15	3.15
3.30	3.30	3.30
3.45	3.45	3.45
4.00	4.00	4.00
4.15	4.15	4.15
4.30	4.30	4.30
4.45	4.45	4.45
5.00	5.00	5.00
5.15	5.15	5.15
5.30	5.30	5.30

Month of_____ Week of_____to_____

THURSDAY /	FRIDAY /	SATURDAY /
8.00	8.00	
8.15	8.15	
8.30	8.30	
8.45	8.45	
9.00	9.00	
9.15	9.15	
9.30	9.30	
9.45	9.45	
10.00	10.00	
10.15	10.15	
10.30	10.30	
10.45	10.45	
11.00	11.00	
11.15	11.15	
11.30	11.30	
11.45	11.45	
12.00	12.00	
12.15	12.15	
12.30	12.30	
12.45	12.45	
1.00	1.00	SUNDAY /
1.15	1.15	
1.30	1.30	
1.45	1.45	
2.00	2.00	
2.15	2.15	
2.30	2.30	
2.45	2.45	
3.00	3.00	
3.15	3.15	
3.30	3.30	
3.45	3.45	
4.00	4.00	
4.15	4.15	
4.30	4.30	
4.45	4.45	
5.00	5.00	
5.15	5.15	
5.30	5.30	

Month of_____ Week of_____to_____

MONDAY /	TUESDAY /	WEDNESDAY /
8.00	8.00	8.00
8.15	8.15	8.15
8.30	8.30	8.30
8.45	8.45	8.45
9.00	9.00	9.00
9.15	9.15	9.15
9.30	9.30	9.30
9.45	9.45	9.45
10.00	10.00	10.00
10.15	10.15	10.15
10.30	10.30	10.30
10.45	10.45	10.45
11.00	11.00	11.00
11.15	11.15	11.15
11.30	11.30	11.30
11.45	11.45	11.45
12.00	12.00	12.00
12.15	12.15	12.15
12.30	12.30	12.30
12.45	12.45	12.45
1.00	1.00	1.00
1.15	1.15	1.15
1.30	1.30	1.30
1.45	1.45	1.45
2.00	2.00	2.00
2.15	2.15	2.15
2.30	2.30	2.30
2.45	2.45	2.45
3.00	3.00	3.00
3.15	3.15	3.15
3.30	3.30	3.30
3.45	3.45	3.45
4.00	4.00	4.00
4.15	4.15	4.15
4.30	4.30	4.30
4.45	4.45	4.45
5.00	5.00	5.00
5.15	5.15	5.15
5.30	5.30	5.30

Month of_____ Week of_____ to_____

THURSDAY /	FRIDAY /	SATURDAY /
8.00	8.00	
8.15	8.15	
8.30	8.30	
8.45	8.45	
9.00	9.00	
9.15	9.15	
9.30	9.30	
9.45	9.45	
10.00	10.00	
10.15	10.15	
10.30	10.30	
10.45	10.45	
11.00	11.00	
11.15	11.15	
11.30	11.30	
11.45	11.45	
12.00	12.00	
12.15	12.15	
12.30	12.30	
12.45	12.45	
1.00	1.00	SUNDAY /
1.15	1.15	
1.30	1.30	
1.45	1.45	
2.00	2.00	
2.15	2.15	
2.30	2.30	
2.45	2.45	
3.00	3.00	
3.15	3.15	
3.30	3.30	
3.45	3.45	
4.00	4.00	
4.15	4.15	
4.30	4.30	
4.45	4.45	
5.00	5.00	
5.15	5.15	
5.30	5.30	

Month of_____ Week of_____to_____

MONDAY /	TUESDAY /	WEDNESDAY /
8.00	8.00	8.00
8.15	8.15	8.15
8.30	8.30	8.30
8.45	8.45	8.45
9.00	9.00	9.00
9.15	9.15	9.15
9.30	9.30	9.30
9.45	9.45	9.45
10.00	10.00	10.00
10.15	10.15	10.15
10.30	10.30	10.30
10.45	10.45	10.45
11.00	11.00	11.00
11.15	11.15	11.15
11.30	11.30	11.30
11.45	11.45	11.45
12.00	12.00	12.00
12.15	12.15	12.15
12.30	12.30	12.30
12.45	12.45	12.45
1.00	1.00	1.00
1.15	1.15	1.15
1.30	1.30	1.30
1.45	1.45	1.45
2.00	2.00	2.00
2.15	2.15	2.15
2.30	2.30	2.30
2.45	2.45	2.45
3.00	3.00	3.00
3.15	3.15	3.15
3.30	3.30	3.30
3.45	3.45	3.45
4.00	4.00	4.00
4.15	4.15	4.15
4.30	4.30	4.30
4.45	4.45	4.45
5.00	5.00	5.00
5.15	5.15	5.15
5.30	5.30	5.30

Month of_____ Week of_____to_____

THURSDAY /	FRIDAY /	SATURDAY /
8.00	8.00	
8.15	8.15	
8.30	8.30	
8.45	8.45	
9.00	9.00	
9.15	9.15	
9.30	9.30	
9.45	9.45	
10.00	10.00	
10.15	10.15	
10.30	10.30	
10.45	10.45	
11.00	11.00	
11.15	11.15	
11.30	11.30	
11.45	11.45	
12.00	12.00	
12.15	12.15	
12.30	12.30	
12.45	12.45	
1.00	1.00	SUNDAY /
1.15	1.15	
1.30	1.30	
1.45	1.45	
2.00	2.00	
2.15	2.15	
2.30	2.30	
2.45	2.45	
3.00	3.00	
3.15	3.15	
3.30	3.30	
3.45	3.45	
4.00	4.00	
4.15	4.15	
4.30	4.30	
4.45	4.45	
5.00	5.00	
5.15	5.15	
5.30	5.30	

Month of_____ Week of_____to_____

MONDAY /	TUESDAY /	WEDNESDAY /
8.00	8.00	8.00
8.15	8.15	8.15
8.30	8.30	8.30
8.45	8.45	8.45
9.00	9.00	9.00
9.15	9.15	9.15
9.30	9.30	9.30
9.45	9.45	9.45
10.00	10.00	10.00
10.15	10.15	10.15
10.30	10.30	10.30
10.45	10.45	10.45
11.00	11.00	11.00
11.15	11.15	11.15
11.30	11.30	11.30
11.45	11.45	11.45
12.00	12.00	12.00
12.15	12.15	12.15
12.30	12.30	12.30
12.45	12.45	12.45
1.00	1.00	1.00
1.15	1.15	1.15
1.30	1.30	1.30
1.45	1.45	1.45
2.00	2.00	2.00
2.15	2.15	2.15
2.30	2.30	2.30
2.45	2.45	2.45
3.00	3.00	3.00
3.15	3.15	3.15
3.30	3.30	3.30
3.45	3.45	3.45
4.00	4.00	4.00
4.15	4.15	4.15
4.30	4.30	4.30
4.45	4.45	4.45
5.00	5.00	5.00
5.15	5.15	5.15
5.30	5.30	5.30

Month of_____ Week of_____to_____

THURSDAY /	FRIDAY /	SATURDAY /
8.00	8.00	
8.15	8.15	
8.30	8.30	
8.45	8.45	
9.00	9.00	
9.15	9.15	
9.30	9.30	
9.45	9.45	
10.00	10.00	
10.15	10.15	
10.30	10.30	
10.45	10.45	
11.00	11.00	
11.15	11.15	
11.30	11.30	
11.45	11.45	
12.00	12.00	
12.15	12.15	
12.30	12.30	
12.45	12.45	
1.00	1.00	SUNDAY /
1.15	1.15	
1.30	1.30	
1.45	1.45	
2.00	2.00	
2.15	2.15	
2.30	2.30	
2.45	2.45	
3.00	3.00	
3.15	3.15	
3.30	3.30	
3.45	3.45	
4.00	4.00	
4.15	4.15	
4.30	4.30	
4.45	4.45	
5.00	5.00	
5.15	5.15	
5.30	5.30	

Month of_____ Week of_____to_____

MONDAY /	TUESDAY /	WEDNESDAY /
8.00	**8.00**	**8.00**
8.15	8.15	8.15
8.30	8.30	8.30
8.45	8.45	8.45
9.00	**9.00**	**9.00**
9.15	9.15	9.15
9.30	9.30	9.30
9.45	9.45	9.45
10.00	**10.00**	**10.00**
10.15	10.15	10.15
10.30	10.30	10.30
10.45	**10.45**	**10.45**
11.00	**11.00**	**11.00**
11.15	11.15	11.15
11.30	11.30	11.30
11.45	11.45	11.45
12.00	**12.00**	**12.00**
12.15	12.15	12.15
12.30	12.30	12.30
12.45	12.45	12.45
1.00	**1.00**	**1.00**
1.15	1.15	1.15
1.30	1.30	1.30
1.45	1.45	1.45
2.00	**2.00**	**2.00**
2.15	2.15	2.15
2.30	2.30	2.30
2.45	2.45	2.45
3.00	**3.00**	**3.00**
3.15	3.15	3.15
3.30	3.30	3.30
3.45	3.45	3.45
4.00	**4.00**	**4.00**
4.15	4.15	4.15
4.30	4.30	4.30
4.45	4.45	4.45
5.00	**5.00**	**5.00**
5.15	5.15	5.15
5.30	5.30	5.30

Month of_____ Week of_____to_____

THURSDAY /	FRIDAY /	SATURDAY /
8.00	8.00	
8.15	8.15	
8.30	8.30	
8.45	8.45	
9.00	9.00	
9.15	9.15	
9.30	9.30	
9.45	9.45	
10.00	10.00	
10.15	10.15	
10.30	10.30	
10.45	10.45	
11.00	11.00	
11.15	11.15	
11.30	11.30	
11.45	11.45	
12.00	12.00	
12.15	12.15	
12.30	12.30	
12.45	12.45	
1.00	1.00	SUNDAY /
1.15	1.15	
1.30	1.30	
1.45	1.45	
2.00	2.00	
2.15	2.15	
2.30	2.30	
2.45	2.45	
3.00	3.00	
3.15	3.15	
3.30	3.30	
3.45	3.45	
4.00	4.00	
4.15	4.15	
4.30	4.30	
4.45	4.45	
5.00	5.00	
5.15	5.15	
5.30	5.30	

Month of_____ Week of_____to_____

MONDAY /	TUESDAY /	WEDNESDAY /
8.00	8.00	8.00
8.15	8.15	8.15
8.30	8.30	8.30
8.45	8.45	8.45
9.00	9.00	9.00
9.15	9.15	9.15
9.30	9.30	9.30
9.45	9.45	9.45
10.00	10.00	10.00
10.15	10.15	10.15
10.30	10.30	10.30
10.45	10.45	10.45
11.00	11.00	11.00
11.15	11.15	11.15
11.30	11.30	11.30
11.45	11.45	11.45
12.00	12.00	12.00
12.15	12.15	12.15
12.30	12.30	12.30
12.45	12.45	12.45
1.00	1.00	1.00
1.15	1.15	1.15
1.30	1.30	1.30
1.45	1.45	1.45
2.00	2.00	2.00
2.15	2.15	2.15
2.30	2.30	2.30
2.45	2.45	2.45
3.00	3.00	3.00
3.15	3.15	3.15
3.30	3.30	3.30
3.45	3.45	3.45
4.00	4.00	4.00
4.15	4.15	4.15
4.30	4.30	4.30
4.45	4.45	4.45
5.00	5.00	5.00
5.15	5.15	5.15
5.30	5.30	5.30

Month of_____ Week of_____to_____

THURSDAY /	FRIDAY /	SATURDAY /
8.00	8.00	
8.15	8.15	
8.30	8.30	
8.45	8.45	
9.00	9.00	
9.15	9.15	
9.30	9.30	
9.45	9.45	
10.00	10.00	
10.15	10.15	
10.30	10.30	
10.45	10.45	
11.00	11.00	
11.15	11.15	
11.30	11.30	
11.45	11.45	
12.00	12.00	
12.15	12.15	
12.30	12.30	
12.45	12.45	
1.00	1.00	SUNDAY /
1.15	1.15	
1.30	1.30	
1.45	1.45	
2.00	2.00	
2.15	2.15	
2.30	2.30	
2.45	2.45	
3.00	3.00	
3.15	3.15	
3.30	3.30	
3.45	3.45	
4.00	4.00	
4.15	4.15	
4.30	4.30	
4.45	4.45	
5.00	5.00	
5.15	5.15	
5.30	5.30	

Month of_____ Week of_____to_____

MONDAY /	TUESDAY /	WEDNESDAY /
8.00	8.00	8.00
8.15	8.15	8.15
8.30	8.30	8.30
8.45	8.45	8.45
9.00	9.00	9.00
9.15	9.15	9.15
9.30	9.30	9.30
9.45	9.45	9.45
10.00	10.00	10.00
10.15	10.15	10.15
10.30	10.30	10.30
10.45	10.45	10.45
11.00	11.00	11.00
11.15	11.15	11.15
11.30	11.30	11.30
11.45	11.45	11.45
12.00	12.00	12.00
12.15	12.15	12.15
12.30	12.30	12.30
12.45	12.45	12.45
1.00	1.00	1.00
1.15	1.15	1.15
1.30	1.30	1.30
1.45	1.45	1.45
2.00	2.00	2.00
2.15	2.15	2.15
2.30	2.30	2.30
2.45	2.45	2.45
3.00	3.00	3.00
3.15	3.15	3.15
3.30	3.30	3.30
3.45	3.45	3.45
4.00	4.00	4.00
4.15	4.15	4.15
4.30	4.30	4.30
4.45	4.45	4.45
5.00	5.00	5.00
5.15	5.15	5.15
5.30	5.30	5.30

Month of_____ Week of_____to_____

THURSDAY /	FRIDAY /	SATURDAY /
8.00	**8.00**	
8.15	8.15	
8.30	8.30	
8.45	8.45	
9.00	**9.00**	
9.15	9.15	
9.30	9.30	
9.45	9.45	
10.00	**10.00**	
10.15	10.15	
10.30	10.30	
10.45	**10.45**	
11.00	**11.00**	
11.15	11.15	
11.30	11.30	
11.45	11.45	
12.00	**12.00**	
12.15	12.15	
12.30	12.30	
12.45	12.45	
1.00	**1.00**	**SUNDAY /**
1.15	1.15	
1.30	1.30	
1.45	1.45	
2.00	**2.00**	
2.15	2.15	
2.30	2.30	
2.45	2.45	
3.00	**3.00**	
3.15	3.15	
3.30	3.30	
3.45	3.45	
4.00	**4.00**	
4.15	4.15	
4.30	4.30	
4.45	4.45	
5.00	**5.00**	
5.15	5.15	
5.30	5.30	

Month of_____ Week of_____to_____

MONDAY /	TUESDAY /	WEDNESDAY /
8.00	8.00	8.00
8.15	8.15	8.15
8.30	8.30	8.30
8.45	8.45	8.45
9.00	9.00	9.00
9.15	9.15	9.15
9.30	9.30	9.30
9.45	9.45	9.45
10.00	10.00	10.00
10.15	10.15	10.15
10.30	10.30	10.30
10.45	10.45	10.45
11.00	11.00	11.00
11.15	11.15	11.15
11.30	11.30	11.30
11.45	11.45	11.45
12.00	12.00	12.00
12.15	12.15	12.15
12.30	12.30	12.30
12.45	12.45	12.45
1.00	1.00	1.00
1.15	1.15	1.15
1.30	1.30	1.30
1.45	1.45	1.45
2.00	2.00	2.00
2.15	2.15	2.15
2.30	2.30	2.30
2.45	2.45	2.45
3.00	3.00	3.00
3.15	3.15	3.15
3.30	3.30	3.30
3.45	3.45	3.45
4.00	4.00	4.00
4.15	4.15	4.15
4.30	4.30	4.30
4.45	4.45	4.45
5.00	5.00	5.00
5.15	5.15	5.15
5.30	5.30	5.30

Month of_____ Week of_____to_____

THURSDAY /	FRIDAY /	SATURDAY /
8.00	8.00	
8.15	8.15	
8.30	8.30	
8.45	8.45	
9.00	9.00	
9.15	9.15	
9.30	9.30	
9.45	9.45	
10.00	10.00	
10.15	10.15	
10.30	10.30	
10.45	10.45	
11.00	11.00	
11.15	11.15	
11.30	11.30	
11.45	11.45	
12.00	12.00	
12.15	12.15	
12.30	12.30	
12.45	12.45	
1.00	1.00	SUNDAY /
1.15	1.15	
1.30	1.30	
1.45	1.45	
2.00	2.00	
2.15	2.15	
2.30	2.30	
2.45	2.45	
3.00	3.00	
3.15	3.15	
3.30	3.30	
3.45	3.45	
4.00	4.00	
4.15	4.15	
4.30	4.30	
4.45	4.45	
5.00	5.00	
5.15	5.15	
5.30	5.30	

Month of_____ Week of_____to_____

MONDAY /	TUESDAY /	WEDNESDAY /
8.00	8.00	8.00
8.15	8.15	8.15
8.30	8.30	8.30
8.45	8.45	8.45
9.00	9.00	9.00
9.15	9.15	9.15
9.30	9.30	9.30
9.45	9.45	9.45
10.00	10.00	10.00
10.15	10.15	10.15
10.30	10.30	10.30
10.45	10.45	10.45
11.00	11.00	11.00
11.15	11.15	11.15
11.30	11.30	11.30
11.45	11.45	11.45
12.00	12.00	12.00
12.15	12.15	12.15
12.30	12.30	12.30
12.45	12.45	12.45
1.00	1.00	1.00
1.15	1.15	1.15
1.30	1.30	1.30
1.45	1.45	1.45
2.00	2.00	2.00
2.15	2.15	2.15
2.30	2.30	2.30
2.45	2.45	2.45
3.00	3.00	3.00
3.15	3.15	3.15
3.30	3.30	3.30
3.45	3.45	3.45
4.00	4.00	4.00
4.15	4.15	4.15
4.30	4.30	4.30
4.45	4.45	4.45
5.00	5.00	5.00
5.15	5.15	5.15
5.30	5.30	5.30

Month of_____ Week of_____to_____

THURSDAY /	FRIDAY /	SATURDAY /
8.00	8.00	
8.15	8.15	
8.30	8.30	
8.45	8.45	
9.00	9.00	
9.15	9.15	
9.30	9.30	
9.45	9.45	
10.00	10.00	
10.15	10.15	
10.30	10.30	
10.45	10.45	
11.00	11.00	
11.15	11.15	
11.30	11.30	
11.45	11.45	
12.00	12.00	
12.15	12.15	
12.30	12.30	
12.45	12.45	
1.00	1.00	SUNDAY /
1.15	1.15	
1.30	1.30	
1.45	1.45	
2.00	2.00	
2.15	2.15	
2.30	2.30	
2.45	2.45	
3.00	3.00	
3.15	3.15	
3.30	3.30	
3.45	3.45	
4.00	4.00	
4.15	4.15	
4.30	4.30	
4.45	4.45	
5.00	5.00	
5.15	5.15	
5.30	5.30	

Month of_____ Week of_____to_____

MONDAY /	TUESDAY /	WEDNESDAY /
8.00	8.00	8.00
8.15	8.15	8.15
8.30	8.30	8.30
8.45	8.45	8.45
9.00	9.00	9.00
9.15	9.15	9.15
9.30	9.30	9.30
9.45	9.45	9.45
10.00	10.00	10.00
10.15	10.15	10.15
10.30	10.30	10.30
10.45	10.45	10.45
11.00	11.00	11.00
11.15	11.15	11.15
11.30	11.30	11.30
11.45	11.45	11.45
12.00	12.00	12.00
12.15	12.15	12.15
12.30	12.30	12.30
12.45	12.45	12.45
1.00	1.00	1.00
1.15	1.15	1.15
1.30	1.30	1.30
1.45	1.45	1.45
2.00	2.00	2.00
2.15	2.15	2.15
2.30	2.30	2.30
2.45	2.45	2.45
3.00	3.00	3.00
3.15	3.15	3.15
3.30	3.30	3.30
3.45	3.45	3.45
4.00	4.00	4.00
4.15	4.15	4.15
4.30	4.30	4.30
4.45	4.45	4.45
5.00	5.00	5.00
5.15	5.15	5.15
5.30	5.30	5.30

Month of_____ Week of_____to_____

THURSDAY /	FRIDAY /	SATURDAY /
8.00	8.00	
8.15	8.15	
8.30	8.30	
8.45	8.45	
9.00	9.00	
9.15	9.15	
9.30	9.30	
9.45	9.45	
10.00	10.00	
10.15	10.15	
10.30	10.30	
10.45	10.45	
11.00	11.00	
11.15	11.15	
11.30	11.30	
11.45	11.45	
12.00	12.00	
12.15	12.15	
12.30	12.30	
12.45	12.45	
1.00	1.00	SUNDAY /
1.15	1.15	
1.30	1.30	
1.45	1.45	
2.00	2.00	
2.15	2.15	
2.30	2.30	
2.45	2.45	
3.00	3.00	
3.15	3.15	
3.30	3.30	
3.45	3.45	
4.00	4.00	
4.15	4.15	
4.30	4.30	
4.45	4.45	
5.00	5.00	
5.15	5.15	
5.30	5.30	

Month of_____ Week of_____to_____

MONDAY /	TUESDAY /	WEDNESDAY /
8.00	8.00	8.00
8.15	8.15	8.15
8.30	8.30	8.30
8.45	8.45	8.45
9.00	9.00	9.00
9.15	9.15	9.15
9.30	9.30	9.30
9.45	9.45	9.45
10.00	10.00	10.00
10.15	10.15	10.15
10.30	10.30	10.30
10.45	10.45	10.45
11.00	11.00	11.00
11.15	11.15	11.15
11.30	11.30	11.30
11.45	11.45	11.45
12.00	12.00	12.00
12.15	12.15	12.15
12.30	12.30	12.30
12.45	12.45	12.45
1.00	1.00	1.00
1.15	1.15	1.15
1.30	1.30	1.30
1.45	1.45	1.45
2.00	2.00	2.00
2.15	2.15	2.15
2.30	2.30	2.30
2.45	2.45	2.45
3.00	3.00	3.00
3.15	3.15	3.15
3.30	3.30	3.30
3.45	3.45	3.45
4.00	4.00	4.00
4.15	4.15	4.15
4.30	4.30	4.30
4.45	4.45	4.45
5.00	5.00	5.00
5.15	5.15	5.15
5.30	5.30	5.30

Month of_____ Week of_____to_____

THURSDAY /	FRIDAY /	SATURDAY /
8.00	8.00	
8.15	8.15	
8.30	8.30	
8.45	8.45	
9.00	9.00	
9.15	9.15	
9.30	9.30	
9.45	9.45	
10.00	10.00	
10.15	10.15	
10.30	10.30	
10.45	10.45	
11.00	11.00	
11.15	11.15	
11.30	11.30	
11.45	11.45	
12.00	12.00	
12.15	12.15	
12.30	12.30	
12.45	12.45	
1.00	1.00	SUNDAY /
1.15	1.15	
1.30	1.30	
1.45	1.45	
2.00	2.00	
2.15	2.15	
2.30	2.30	
2.45	2.45	
3.00	3.00	
3.15	3.15	
3.30	3.30	
3.45	3.45	
4.00	4.00	
4.15	4.15	
4.30	4.30	
4.45	4.45	
5.00	5.00	
5.15	5.15	
5.30	5.30	

Month of_____ Week of_____to_____

MONDAY /	TUESDAY /	WEDNESDAY /
8.00	8.00	8.00
8.15	8.15	8.15
8.30	8.30	8.30
8.45	8.45	8.45
9.00	9.00	9.00
9.15	9.15	9.15
9.30	9.30	9.30
9.45	9.45	9.45
10.00	10.00	10.00
10.15	10.15	10.15
10.30	10.30	10.30
10.45	10.45	10.45
11.00	11.00	11.00
11.15	11.15	11.15
11.30	11.30	11.30
11.45	11.45	11.45
12.00	12.00	12.00
12.15	12.15	12.15
12.30	12.30	12.30
12.45	12.45	12.45
1.00	1.00	1.00
1.15	1.15	1.15
1.30	1.30	1.30
1.45	1.45	1.45
2.00	2.00	2.00
2.15	2.15	2.15
2.30	2.30	2.30
2.45	2.45	2.45
3.00	3.00	3.00
3.15	3.15	3.15
3.30	3.30	3.30
3.45	3.45	3.45
4.00	4.00	4.00
4.15	4.15	4.15
4.30	4.30	4.30
4.45	4.45	4.45
5.00	5.00	5.00
5.15	5.15	5.15
5.30	5.30	5.30

Month of_____ Week of_____to_____

THURSDAY /	FRIDAY /	SATURDAY /
8.00	8.00	
8.15	8.15	
8.30	8.30	
8.45	8.45	
9.00	9.00	
9.15	9.15	
9.30	9.30	
9.45	9.45	
10.00	10.00	
10.15	10.15	
10.30	10.30	
10.45	10.45	
11.00	11.00	
11.15	11.15	
11.30	11.30	
11.45	11.45	
12.00	12.00	
12.15	12.15	
12.30	12.30	
12.45	12.45	
1.00	1.00	SUNDAY /
1.15	1.15	
1.30	1.30	
1.45	1.45	
2.00	2.00	
2.15	2.15	
2.30	2.30	
2.45	2.45	
3.00	3.00	
3.15	3.15	
3.30	3.30	
3.45	3.45	
4.00	4.00	
4.15	4.15	
4.30	4.30	
4.45	4.45	
5.00	5.00	
5.15	5.15	
5.30	5.30	

Month of_____ Week of_____to_____

MONDAY /	TUESDAY /	WEDNESDAY /
8.00	8.00	8.00
8.15	8.15	8.15
8.30	8.30	8.30
8.45	8.45	8.45
9.00	9.00	9.00
9.15	9.15	9.15
9.30	9.30	9.30
9.45	9.45	9.45
10.00	10.00	10.00
10.15	10.15	10.15
10.30	10.30	10.30
10.45	10.45	10.45
11.00	11.00	11.00
11.15	11.15	11.15
11.30	11.30	11.30
11.45	11.45	11.45
12.00	12.00	12.00
12.15	12.15	12.15
12.30	12.30	12.30
12.45	12.45	12.45
1.00	1.00	1.00
1.15	1.15	1.15
1.30	1.30	1.30
1.45	1.45	1.45
2.00	2.00	2.00
2.15	2.15	2.15
2.30	2.30	2.30
2.45	2.45	2.45
3.00	3.00	3.00
3.15	3.15	3.15
3.30	3.30	3.30
3.45	3.45	3.45
4.00	4.00	4.00
4.15	4.15	4.15
4.30	4.30	4.30
4.45	4.45	4.45
5.00	5.00	5.00
5.15	5.15	5.15
5.30	5.30	5.30

Month of_____ Week of_____to_____

THURSDAY /	FRIDAY /	SATURDAY /
8.00	8.00	
8.15	8.15	
8.30	8.30	
8.45	8.45	
9.00	9.00	
9.15	9.15	
9.30	9.30	
9.45	9.45	
10.00	10.00	
10.15	10.15	
10.30	10.30	
10.45	10.45	
11.00	11.00	
11.15	11.15	
11.30	11.30	
11.45	11.45	
12.00	12.00	
12.15	12.15	
12.30	12.30	
12.45	12.45	
1.00	1.00	SUNDAY /
1.15	1.15	
1.30	1.30	
1.45	1.45	
2.00	2.00	
2.15	2.15	
2.30	2.30	
2.45	2.45	
3.00	3.00	
3.15	3.15	
3.30	3.30	
3.45	3.45	
4.00	4.00	
4.15	4.15	
4.30	4.30	
4.45	4.45	
5.00	5.00	
5.15	5.15	
5.30	5.30	

Month of_____ Week of_____to_____

MONDAY /	TUESDAY /	WEDNESDAY /
8.00	8.00	8.00
8.15	8.15	8.15
8.30	8.30	8.30
8.45	8.45	8.45
9.00	9.00	9.00
9.15	9.15	9.15
9.30	9.30	9.30
9.45	9.45	9.45
10.00	10.00	10.00
10.15	10.15	10.15
10.30	10.30	10.30
10.45	10.45	10.45
11.00	11.00	11.00
11.15	11.15	11.15
11.30	11.30	11.30
11.45	11.45	11.45
12.00	12.00	12.00
12.15	12.15	12.15
12.30	12.30	12.30
12.45	12.45	12.45
1.00	1.00	1.00
1.15	1.15	1.15
1.30	1.30	1.30
1.45	1.45	1.45
2.00	2.00	2.00
2.15	2.15	2.15
2.30	2.30	2.30
2.45	2.45	2.45
3.00	3.00	3.00
3.15	3.15	3.15
3.30	3.30	3.30
3.45	3.45	3.45
4.00	4.00	4.00
4.15	4.15	4.15
4.30	4.30	4.30
4.45	4.45	4.45
5.00	5.00	5.00
5.15	5.15	5.15
5.30	5.30	5.30

Month of_____ Week of_____to_____

THURSDAY /	FRIDAY /	SATURDAY /
8.00	8.00	
8.15	8.15	
8.30	8.30	
8.45	8.45	
9.00	9.00	
9.15	9.15	
9.30	9.30	
9.45	9.45	
10.00	10.00	
10.15	10.15	
10.30	10.30	
10.45	10.45	
11.00	11.00	
11.15	11.15	
11.30	11.30	
11.45	11.45	
12.00	12.00	
12.15	12.15	
12.30	12.30	
12.45	12.45	
1.00	1.00	SUNDAY /
1.15	1.15	
1.30	1.30	
1.45	1.45	
2.00	2.00	
2.15	2.15	
2.30	2.30	
2.45	2.45	
3.00	3.00	
3.15	3.15	
3.30	3.30	
3.45	3.45	
4.00	4.00	
4.15	4.15	
4.30	4.30	
4.45	4.45	
5.00	5.00	
5.15	5.15	
5.30	5.30	

Month of_____ Week of_____to_____

MONDAY /	TUESDAY /	WEDNESDAY /
8.00	8.00	8.00
8.15	8.15	8.15
8.30	8.30	8.30
8.45	8.45	8.45
9.00	9.00	9.00
9.15	9.15	9.15
9.30	9.30	9.30
9.45	9.45	9.45
10.00	10.00	10.00
10.15	10.15	10.15
10.30	10.30	10.30
10.45	10.45	10.45
11.00	11.00	11.00
11.15	11.15	11.15
11.30	11.30	11.30
11.45	11.45	11.45
12.00	12.00	12.00
12.15	12.15	12.15
12.30	12.30	12.30
12.45	12.45	12.45
1.00	1.00	1.00
1.15	1.15	1.15
1.30	1.30	1.30
1.45	1.45	1.45
2.00	2.00	2.00
2.15	2.15	2.15
2.30	2.30	2.30
2.45	2.45	2.45
3.00	3.00	3.00
3.15	3.15	3.15
3.30	3.30	3.30
3.45	3.45	3.45
4.00	4.00	4.00
4.15	4.15	4.15
4.30	4.30	4.30
4.45	4.45	4.45
5.00	5.00	5.00
5.15	5.15	5.15
5.30	5.30	5.30

Month of_____ Week of_____to_____

THURSDAY /	FRIDAY /	SATURDAY /
8.00	8.00	
8.15	8.15	
8.30	8.30	
8.45	8.45	
9.00	9.00	
9.15	9.15	
9.30	9.30	
9.45	9.45	
10.00	10.00	
10.15	10.15	
10.30	10.30	
10.45	10.45	
11.00	11.00	
11.15	11.15	
11.30	11.30	
11.45	11.45	
12.00	12.00	
12.15	12.15	
12.30	12.30	
12.45	12.45	
1.00	1.00	SUNDAY /
1.15	1.15	
1.30	1.30	
1.45	1.45	
2.00	2.00	
2.15	2.15	
2.30	2.30	
2.45	2.45	
3.00	3.00	
3.15	3.15	
3.30	3.30	
3.45	3.45	
4.00	4.00	
4.15	4.15	
4.30	4.30	
4.45	4.45	
5.00	5.00	
5.15	5.15	
5.30	5.30	

Month of_____ Week of_____to_____

MONDAY /	TUESDAY /	WEDNESDAY /
8.00	8.00	8.00
8.15	8.15	8.15
8.30	8.30	8.30
8.45	8.45	8.45
9.00	9.00	9.00
9.15	9.15	9.15
9.30	9.30	9.30
9.45	9.45	9.45
10.00	10.00	10.00
10.15	10.15	10.15
10.30	10.30	10.30
10.45	10.45	10.45
11.00	11.00	11.00
11.15	11.15	11.15
11.30	11.30	11.30
11.45	11.45	11.45
12.00	12.00	12.00
12.15	12.15	12.15
12.30	12.30	12.30
12.45	12.45	12.45
1.00	1.00	1.00
1.15	1.15	1.15
1.30	1.30	1.30
1.45	1.45	1.45
2.00	2.00	2.00
2.15	2.15	2.15
2.30	2.30	2.30
2.45	2.45	2.45
3.00	3.00	3.00
3.15	3.15	3.15
3.30	3.30	3.30
3.45	3.45	3.45
4.00	4.00	4.00
4.15	4.15	4.15
4.30	4.30	4.30
4.45	4.45	4.45
5.00	5.00	5.00
5.15	5.15	5.15
5.30	5.30	5.30

Month of_____ Week of_____to_____

THURSDAY /	FRIDAY /	SATURDAY /
8.00	8.00	
8.15	8.15	
8.30	8.30	
8.45	8.45	
9.00	9.00	
9.15	9.15	
9.30	9.30	
9.45	9.45	
10.00	10.00	
10.15	10.15	
10.30	10.30	
10.45	10.45	
11.00	11.00	
11.15	11.15	
11.30	11.30	
11.45	11.45	
12.00	12.00	
12.15	12.15	
12.30	12.30	
12.45	12.45	
1.00	1.00	SUNDAY /
1.15	1.15	
1.30	1.30	
1.45	1.45	
2.00	2.00	
2.15	2.15	
2.30	2.30	
2.45	2.45	
3.00	3.00	
3.15	3.15	
3.30	3.30	
3.45	3.45	
4.00	4.00	
4.15	4.15	
4.30	4.30	
4.45	4.45	
5.00	5.00	
5.15	5.15	
5.30	5.30	

Month of_____ Week of_____to_____

MONDAY /	TUESDAY /	WEDNESDAY /
8.00	**8.00**	**8.00**
8.15	8.15	8.15
8.30	8.30	8.30
8.45	8.45	8.45
9.00	**9.00**	**9.00**
9.15	9.15	9.15
9.30	9.30	9.30
9.45	9.45	9.45
10.00	**10.00**	**10.00**
10.15	10.15	10.15
10.30	10.30	10.30
10.45	**10.45**	**10.45**
11.00	**11.00**	**11.00**
11.15	11.15	11.15
11.30	11.30	11.30
11.45	11.45	11.45
12.00	**12.00**	**12.00**
12.15	12.15	12.15
12.30	12.30	12.30
12.45	12.45	12.45
1.00	**1.00**	**1.00**
1.15	1.15	1.15
1.30	1.30	1.30
1.45	1.45	1.45
2.00	**2.00**	**2.00**
2.15	2.15	2.15
2.30	2.30	2.30
2.45	2.45	2.45
3.00	**3.00**	**3.00**
3.15	3.15	3.15
3.30	3.30	3.30
3.45	3.45	3.45
4.00	**4.00**	**4.00**
4.15	4.15	4.15
4.30	4.30	4.30
4.45	4.45	4.45
5.00	**5.00**	**5.00**
5.15	5.15	5.15
5.30	5.30	5.30

Month of_____ Week of_____to_____

THURSDAY /	FRIDAY /	SATURDAY /
8.00	8.00	
8.15	8.15	
8.30	8.30	
8.45	8.45	
9.00	9.00	
9.15	9.15	
9.30	9.30	
9.45	9.45	
10.00	10.00	
10.15	10.15	
10.30	10.30	
10.45	10.45	
11.00	11.00	
11.15	11.15	
11.30	11.30	
11.45	11.45	
12.00	12.00	
12.15	12.15	
12.30	12.30	
12.45	12.45	
1.00	1.00	SUNDAY /
1.15	1.15	
1.30	1.30	
1.45	1.45	
2.00	2.00	
2.15	2.15	
2.30	2.30	
2.45	2.45	
3.00	3.00	
3.15	3.15	
3.30	3.30	
3.45	3.45	
4.00	4.00	
4.15	4.15	
4.30	4.30	
4.45	4.45	
5.00	5.00	
5.15	5.15	
5.30	5.30	

Month of_____ Week of_____to_____

MONDAY /	TUESDAY /	WEDNESDAY /
8.00	8.00	8.00
8.15	8.15	8.15
8.30	8.30	8.30
8.45	8.45	8.45
9.00	9.00	9.00
9.15	9.15	9.15
9.30	9.30	9.30
9.45	9.45	9.45
10.00	10.00	10.00
10.15	10.15	10.15
10.30	10.30	10.30
10.45	10.45	10.45
11.00	11.00	11.00
11.15	11.15	11.15
11.30	11.30	11.30
11.45	11.45	11.45
12.00	12.00	12.00
12.15	12.15	12.15
12.30	12.30	12.30
12.45	12.45	12.45
1.00	1.00	1.00
1.15	1.15	1.15
1.30	1.30	1.30
1.45	1.45	1.45
2.00	2.00	2.00
2.15	2.15	2.15
2.30	2.30	2.30
2.45	2.45	2.45
3.00	3.00	3.00
3.15	3.15	3.15
3.30	3.30	3.30
3.45	3.45	3.45
4.00	4.00	4.00
4.15	4.15	4.15
4.30	4.30	4.30
4.45	4.45	4.45
5.00	5.00	5.00
5.15	5.15	5.15
5.30	5.30	5.30

Month of_____ Week of_____to_____

THURSDAY /	FRIDAY /	SATURDAY /
8.00	8.00	
8.15	8.15	
8.30	8.30	
8.45	8.45	
9.00	9.00	
9.15	9.15	
9.30	9.30	
9.45	9.45	
10.00	10.00	
10.15	10.15	
10.30	10.30	
10.45	10.45	
11.00	11.00	
11.15	11.15	
11.30	11.30	
11.45	11.45	
12.00	12.00	
12.15	12.15	
12.30	12.30	
12.45	12.45	
1.00	1.00	SUNDAY /
1.15	1.15	
1.30	1.30	
1.45	1.45	
2.00	2.00	
2.15	2.15	
2.30	2.30	
2.45	2.45	
3.00	3.00	
3.15	3.15	
3.30	3.30	
3.45	3.45	
4.00	4.00	
4.15	4.15	
4.30	4.30	
4.45	4.45	
5.00	5.00	
5.15	5.15	
5.30	5.30	

Month of_____ Week of_____to_____

MONDAY /	TUESDAY /	WEDNESDAY /
8.00	8.00	8.00
8.15	8.15	8.15
8.30	8.30	8.30
8.45	8.45	8.45
9.00	9.00	9.00
9.15	9.15	9.15
9.30	9.30	9.30
9.45	9.45	9.45
10.00	10.00	10.00
10.15	10.15	10.15
10.30	10.30	10.30
10.45	10.45	10.45
11.00	11.00	11.00
11.15	11.15	11.15
11.30	11.30	11.30
11.45	11.45	11.45
12.00	12.00	12.00
12.15	12.15	12.15
12.30	12.30	12.30
12.45	12.45	12.45
1.00	1.00	1.00
1.15	1.15	1.15
1.30	1.30	1.30
1.45	1.45	1.45
2.00	2.00	2.00
2.15	2.15	2.15
2.30	2.30	2.30
2.45	2.45	2.45
3.00	3.00	3.00
3.15	3.15	3.15
3.30	3.30	3.30
3.45	3.45	3.45
4.00	4.00	4.00
4.15	4.15	4.15
4.30	4.30	4.30
4.45	4.45	4.45
5.00	5.00	5.00
5.15	5.15	5.15
5.30	5.30	5.30

Month of_____ Week of_____to_____

THURSDAY /	FRIDAY /	SATURDAY /
8.00	8.00	
8.15	8.15	
8.30	8.30	
8.45	8.45	
9.00	9.00	
9.15	9.15	
9.30	9.30	
9.45	9.45	
10.00	10.00	
10.15	10.15	
10.30	10.30	
10.45	10.45	
11.00	11.00	
11.15	11.15	
11.30	11.30	
11.45	11.45	
12.00	12.00	
12.15	12.15	
12.30	12.30	
12.45	12.45	
1.00	1.00	SUNDAY /
1.15	1.15	
1.30	1.30	
1.45	1.45	
2.00	2.00	
2.15	2.15	
2.30	2.30	
2.45	2.45	
3.00	3.00	
3.15	3.15	
3.30	3.30	
3.45	3.45	
4.00	4.00	
4.15	4.15	
4.30	4.30	
4.45	4.45	
5.00	5.00	
5.15	5.15	
5.30	5.30	

Month of_____ Week of_____to_____

MONDAY /	TUESDAY /	WEDNESDAY /
8.00	8.00	8.00
8.15	8.15	8.15
8.30	8.30	8.30
8.45	8.45	8.45
9.00	9.00	9.00
9.15	9.15	9.15
9.30	9.30	9.30
9.45	9.45	9.45
10.00	10.00	10.00
10.15	10.15	10.15
10.30	10.30	10.30
10.45	10.45	10.45
11.00	11.00	11.00
11.15	11.15	11.15
11.30	11.30	11.30
11.45	11.45	11.45
12.00	12.00	12.00
12.15	12.15	12.15
12.30	12.30	12.30
12.45	12.45	12.45
1.00	1.00	1.00
1.15	1.15	1.15
1.30	1.30	1.30
1.45	1.45	1.45
2.00	2.00	2.00
2.15	2.15	2.15
2.30	2.30	2.30
2.45	2.45	2.45
3.00	3.00	3.00
3.15	3.15	3.15
3.30	3.30	3.30
3.45	3.45	3.45
4.00	4.00	4.00
4.15	4.15	4.15
4.30	4.30	4.30
4.45	4.45	4.45
5.00	5.00	5.00
5.15	5.15	5.15
5.30	5.30	5.30

Month of_____ Week of_____to_____

THURSDAY /	FRIDAY /	SATURDAY /
8.00	8.00	
8.15	8.15	
8.30	8.30	
8.45	8.45	
9.00	9.00	
9.15	9.15	
9.30	9.30	
9.45	9.45	
10.00	10.00	
10.15	10.15	
10.30	10.30	
10.45	10.45	
11.00	11.00	
11.15	11.15	
11.30	11.30	
11.45	11.45	
12.00	12.00	
12.15	12.15	
12.30	12.30	
12.45	12.45	
1.00	1.00	SUNDAY /
1.15	1.15	
1.30	1.30	
1.45	1.45	
2.00	2.00	
2.15	2.15	
2.30	2.30	
2.45	2.45	
3.00	3.00	
3.15	3.15	
3.30	3.30	
3.45	3.45	
4.00	4.00	
4.15	4.15	
4.30	4.30	
4.45	4.45	
5.00	5.00	
5.15	5.15	
5.30	5.30	

Month of_____ Week of_____to_____

MONDAY /	TUESDAY /	WEDNESDAY /
8.00	8.00	8.00
8.15	8.15	8.15
8.30	8.30	8.30
8.45	8.45	8.45
9.00	9.00	9.00
9.15	9.15	9.15
9.30	9.30	9.30
9.45	9.45	9.45
10.00	10.00	10.00
10.15	10.15	10.15
10.30	10.30	10.30
10.45	10.45	10.45
11.00	11.00	11.00
11.15	11.15	11.15
11.30	11.30	11.30
11.45	11.45	11.45
12.00	12.00	12.00
12.15	12.15	12.15
12.30	12.30	12.30
12.45	12.45	12.45
1.00	1.00	1.00
1.15	1.15	1.15
1.30	1.30	1.30
1.45	1.45	1.45
2.00	2.00	2.00
2.15	2.15	2.15
2.30	2.30	2.30
2.45	2.45	2.45
3.00	3.00	3.00
3.15	3.15	3.15
3.30	3.30	3.30
3.45	3.45	3.45
4.00	4.00	4.00
4.15	4.15	4.15
4.30	4.30	4.30
4.45	4.45	4.45
5.00	5.00	5.00
5.15	5.15	5.15
5.30	5.30	5.30

Month of_____ Week of_____to_____

THURSDAY /	FRIDAY /	SATURDAY /
8.00	8.00	
8.15	8.15	
8.30	8.30	
8.45	8.45	
9.00	9.00	
9.15	9.15	
9.30	9.30	
9.45	9.45	
10.00	10.00	
10.15	10.15	
10.30	10.30	
10.45	10.45	
11.00	11.00	
11.15	11.15	
11.30	11.30	
11.45	11.45	
12.00	12.00	
12.15	12.15	
12.30	12.30	
12.45	12.45	
1.00	1.00	SUNDAY /
1.15	1.15	
1.30	1.30	
1.45	1.45	
2.00	2.00	
2.15	2.15	
2.30	2.30	
2.45	2.45	
3.00	3.00	
3.15	3.15	
3.30	3.30	
3.45	3.45	
4.00	4.00	
4.15	4.15	
4.30	4.30	
4.45	4.45	
5.00	5.00	
5.15	5.15	
5.30	5.30	

Month of_____ Week of_____to_____

MONDAY /	TUESDAY /	WEDNESDAY /
8.00	**8.00**	**8.00**
8.15	8.15	8.15
8.30	8.30	8.30
8.45	8.45	8.45
9.00	**9.00**	**9.00**
9.15	9.15	9.15
9.30	9.30	9.30
9.45	9.45	9.45
10.00	**10.00**	**10.00**
10.15	10.15	10.15
10.30	10.30	10.30
10.45	**10.45**	**10.45**
11.00	**11.00**	**11.00**
11.15	11.15	11.15
11.30	11.30	11.30
11.45	11.45	11.45
12.00	**12.00**	**12.00**
12.15	12.15	12.15
12.30	12.30	12.30
12.45	12.45	12.45
1.00	**1.00**	**1.00**
1.15	1.15	1.15
1.30	1.30	1.30
1.45	1.45	1.45
2.00	**2.00**	**2.00**
2.15	2.15	2.15
2.30	2.30	2.30
2.45	2.45	2.45
3.00	**3.00**	**3.00**
3.15	3.15	3.15
3.30	3.30	3.30
3.45	3.45	3.45
4.00	**4.00**	**4.00**
4.15	4.15	4.15
4.30	4.30	4.30
4.45	4.45	4.45
5.00	**5.00**	**5.00**
5.15	5.15	5.15
5.30	5.30	5.30

Month of_____ Week of_____to_____

THURSDAY /	FRIDAY /	SATURDAY /
8.00	8.00	
8.15	8.15	
8.30	8.30	
8.45	8.45	
9.00	9.00	
9.15	9.15	
9.30	9.30	
9.45	9.45	
10.00	10.00	
10.15	10.15	
10.30	10.30	
10.45	10.45	
11.00	11.00	
11.15	11.15	
11.30	11.30	
11.45	11.45	
12.00	12.00	
12.15	12.15	
12.30	12.30	
12.45	12.45	
1.00	1.00	SUNDAY /
1.15	1.15	
1.30	1.30	
1.45	1.45	
2.00	2.00	
2.15	2.15	
2.30	2.30	
2.45	2.45	
3.00	3.00	
3.15	3.15	
3.30	3.30	
3.45	3.45	
4.00	4.00	
4.15	4.15	
4.30	4.30	
4.45	4.45	
5.00	5.00	
5.15	5.15	
5.30	5.30	

Month of_____ Week of_____to_____

MONDAY /	TUESDAY /	WEDNESDAY /
8.00	8.00	8.00
8.15	8.15	8.15
8.30	8.30	8.30
8.45	8.45	8.45
9.00	9.00	9.00
9.15	9.15	9.15
9.30	9.30	9.30
9.45	9.45	9.45
10.00	10.00	10.00
10.15	10.15	10.15
10.30	10.30	10.30
10.45	10.45	10.45
11.00	11.00	11.00
11.15	11.15	11.15
11.30	11.30	11.30
11.45	11.45	11.45
12.00	12.00	12.00
12.15	12.15	12.15
12.30	12.30	12.30
12.45	12.45	12.45
1.00	1.00	1.00
1.15	1.15	1.15
1.30	1.30	1.30
1.45	1.45	1.45
2.00	2.00	2.00
2.15	2.15	2.15
2.30	2.30	2.30
2.45	2.45	2.45
3.00	3.00	3.00
3.15	3.15	3.15
3.30	3.30	3.30
3.45	3.45	3.45
4.00	4.00	4.00
4.15	4.15	4.15
4.30	4.30	4.30
4.45	4.45	4.45
5.00	5.00	5.00
5.15	5.15	5.15
5.30	5.30	5.30

Month of_____ Week of_____to_____

THURSDAY /	FRIDAY /	SATURDAY /
8.00	8.00	
8.15	8.15	
8.30	8.30	
8.45	8.45	
9.00	9.00	
9.15	9.15	
9.30	9.30	
9.45	9.45	
10.00	10.00	
10.15	10.15	
10.30	10.30	
10.45	10.45	
11.00	11.00	
11.15	11.15	
11.30	11.30	
11.45	11.45	
12.00	12.00	
12.15	12.15	
12.30	12.30	
12.45	12.45	
1.00	1.00	SUNDAY /
1.15	1.15	
1.30	1.30	
1.45	1.45	
2.00	2.00	
2.15	2.15	
2.30	2.30	
2.45	2.45	
3.00	3.00	
3.15	3.15	
3.30	3.30	
3.45	3.45	
4.00	4.00	
4.15	4.15	
4.30	4.30	
4.45	4.45	
5.00	5.00	
5.15	5.15	
5.30	5.30	

Month of_____ Week of_____to_____

MONDAY /	TUESDAY /	WEDNESDAY /
8.00	8.00	8.00
8.15	8.15	8.15
8.30	8.30	8.30
8.45	8.45	8.45
9.00	9.00	9.00
9.15	9.15	9.15
9.30	9.30	9.30
9.45	9.45	9.45
10.00	10.00	10.00
10.15	10.15	10.15
10.30	10.30	10.30
10.45	10.45	10.45
11.00	11.00	11.00
11.15	11.15	11.15
11.30	11.30	11.30
11.45	11.45	11.45
12.00	12.00	12.00
12.15	12.15	12.15
12.30	12.30	12.30
12.45	12.45	12.45
1.00	1.00	1.00
1.15	1.15	1.15
1.30	1.30	1.30
1.45	1.45	1.45
2.00	2.00	2.00
2.15	2.15	2.15
2.30	2.30	2.30
2.45	2.45	2.45
3.00	3.00	3.00
3.15	3.15	3.15
3.30	3.30	3.30
3.45	3.45	3.45
4.00	4.00	4.00
4.15	4.15	4.15
4.30	4.30	4.30
4.45	4.45	4.45
5.00	5.00	5.00
5.15	5.15	5.15
5.30	5.30	5.30

Month of_____ Week of_____to_____

THURSDAY /	FRIDAY /	SATURDAY /
8.00	8.00	
8.15	8.15	
8.30	8.30	
8.45	8.45	
9.00	9.00	
9.15	9.15	
9.30	9.30	
9.45	9.45	
10.00	10.00	
10.15	10.15	
10.30	10.30	
10.45	10.45	
11.00	11.00	
11.15	11.15	
11.30	11.30	
11.45	11.45	
12.00	12.00	
12.15	12.15	
12.30	12.30	
12.45	12.45	
1.00	1.00	SUNDAY /
1.15	1.15	
1.30	1.30	
1.45	1.45	
2.00	2.00	
2.15	2.15	
2.30	2.30	
2.45	2.45	
3.00	3.00	
3.15	3.15	
3.30	3.30	
3.45	3.45	
4.00	4.00	
4.15	4.15	
4.30	4.30	
4.45	4.45	
5.00	5.00	
5.15	5.15	
5.30	5.30	

Month of_____ Week of_____to_____

MONDAY /	TUESDAY /	WEDNESDAY /
8.00	8.00	8.00
8.15	8.15	8.15
8.30	8.30	8.30
8.45	8.45	8.45
9.00	9.00	9.00
9.15	9.15	9.15
9.30	9.30	9.30
9.45	9.45	9.45
10.00	10.00	10.00
10.15	10.15	10.15
10.30	10.30	10.30
10.45	10.45	10.45
11.00	11.00	11.00
11.15	11.15	11.15
11.30	11.30	11.30
11.45	11.45	11.45
12.00	12.00	12.00
12.15	12.15	12.15
12.30	12.30	12.30
12.45	12.45	12.45
1.00	1.00	1.00
1.15	1.15	1.15
1.30	1.30	1.30
1.45	1.45	1.45
2.00	2.00	2.00
2.15	2.15	2.15
2.30	2.30	2.30
2.45	2.45	2.45
3.00	3.00	3.00
3.15	3.15	3.15
3.30	3.30	3.30
3.45	3.45	3.45
4.00	4.00	4.00
4.15	4.15	4.15
4.30	4.30	4.30
4.45	4.45	4.45
5.00	5.00	5.00
5.15	5.15	5.15
5.30	5.30	5.30

Month of_____ Week of_____to_____

THURSDAY /	FRIDAY /	SATURDAY /
8.00	8.00	
8.15	8.15	
8.30	8.30	
8.45	8.45	
9.00	9.00	
9.15	9.15	
9.30	9.30	
9.45	9.45	
10.00	10.00	
10.15	10.15	
10.30	10.30	
10.45	10.45	
11.00	11.00	
11.15	11.15	
11.30	11.30	
11.45	11.45	
12.00	12.00	
12.15	12.15	
12.30	12.30	
12.45	12.45	
1.00	1.00	SUNDAY /
1.15	1.15	
1.30	1.30	
1.45	1.45	
2.00	2.00	
2.15	2.15	
2.30	2.30	
2.45	2.45	
3.00	3.00	
3.15	3.15	
3.30	3.30	
3.45	3.45	
4.00	4.00	
4.15	4.15	
4.30	4.30	
4.45	4.45	
5.00	5.00	
5.15	5.15	
5.30	5.30	

Month of_____ Week of_____to_____

MONDAY /	TUESDAY /	WEDNESDAY /
8.00	8.00	8.00
8.15	8.15	8.15
8.30	8.30	8.30
8.45	8.45	8.45
9.00	9.00	9.00
9.15	9.15	9.15
9.30	9.30	9.30
9.45	9.45	9.45
10.00	10.00	10.00
10.15	10.15	10.15
10.30	10.30	10.30
10.45	10.45	10.45
11.00	11.00	11.00
11.15	11.15	11.15
11.30	11.30	11.30
11.45	11.45	11.45
12.00	12.00	12.00
12.15	12.15	12.15
12.30	12.30	12.30
12.45	12.45	12.45
1.00	1.00	1.00
1.15	1.15	1.15
1.30	1.30	1.30
1.45	1.45	1.45
2.00	2.00	2.00
2.15	2.15	2.15
2.30	2.30	2.30
2.45	2.45	2.45
3.00	3.00	3.00
3.15	3.15	3.15
3.30	3.30	3.30
3.45	3.45	3.45
4.00	4.00	4.00
4.15	4.15	4.15
4.30	4.30	4.30
4.45	4.45	4.45
5.00	5.00	5.00
5.15	5.15	5.15
5.30	5.30	5.30

Month of_____ Week of_____to_____

THURSDAY /	FRIDAY /	SATURDAY /
8.00	8.00	
8.15	8.15	
8.30	8.30	
8.45	8.45	
9.00	9.00	
9.15	9.15	
9.30	9.30	
9.45	9.45	
10.00	10.00	
10.15	10.15	
10.30	10.30	
10.45	10.45	
11.00	11.00	
11.15	11.15	
11.30	11.30	
11.45	11.45	
12.00	12.00	
12.15	12.15	
12.30	12.30	
12.45	12.45	
1.00	1.00	SUNDAY /
1.15	1.15	
1.30	1.30	
1.45	1.45	
2.00	2.00	
2.15	2.15	
2.30	2.30	
2.45	2.45	
3.00	3.00	
3.15	3.15	
3.30	3.30	
3.45	3.45	
4.00	4.00	
4.15	4.15	
4.30	4.30	
4.45	4.45	
5.00	5.00	
5.15	5.15	
5.30	5.30	

Month of_____ Week of_____to_____

MONDAY /	TUESDAY /	WEDNESDAY /
8.00	8.00	8.00
8.15	8.15	8.15
8.30	8.30	8.30
8.45	8.45	8.45
9.00	9.00	9.00
9.15	9.15	9.15
9.30	9.30	9.30
9.45	9.45	9.45
10.00	10.00	10.00
10.15	10.15	10.15
10.30	10.30	10.30
10.45	10.45	10.45
11.00	11.00	11.00
11.15	11.15	11.15
11.30	11.30	11.30
11.45	11.45	11.45
12.00	12.00	12.00
12.15	12.15	12.15
12.30	12.30	12.30
12.45	12.45	12.45
1.00	1.00	1.00
1.15	1.15	1.15
1.30	1.30	1.30
1.45	1.45	1.45
2.00	2.00	2.00
2.15	2.15	2.15
2.30	2.30	2.30
2.45	2.45	2.45
3.00	3.00	3.00
3.15	3.15	3.15
3.30	3.30	3.30
3.45	3.45	3.45
4.00	4.00	4.00
4.15	4.15	4.15
4.30	4.30	4.30
4.45	4.45	4.45
5.00	5.00	5.00
5.15	5.15	5.15
5.30	5.30	5.30

Month of_____ Week of_____to_____

THURSDAY /	FRIDAY /	SATURDAY /
8.00	8.00	
8.15	8.15	
8.30	8.30	
8.45	8.45	
9.00	9.00	
9.15	9.15	
9.30	9.30	
9.45	9.45	
10.00	10.00	
10.15	10.15	
10.30	10.30	
10.45	10.45	
11.00	11.00	
11.15	11.15	
11.30	11.30	
11.45	11.45	
12.00	12.00	
12.15	12.15	
12.30	12.30	
12.45	12.45	
1.00	1.00	SUNDAY /
1.15	1.15	
1.30	1.30	
1.45	1.45	
2.00	2.00	
2.15	2.15	
2.30	2.30	
2.45	2.45	
3.00	3.00	
3.15	3.15	
3.30	3.30	
3.45	3.45	
4.00	4.00	
4.15	4.15	
4.30	4.30	
4.45	4.45	
5.00	5.00	
5.15	5.15	
5.30	5.30	

Month of_____ Week of_____ to_____

MONDAY /	TUESDAY /	WEDNESDAY /
8.00	8.00	8.00
8.15	8.15	8.15
8.30	8.30	8.30
8.45	8.45	8.45
9.00	9.00	9.00
9.15	9.15	9.15
9.30	9.30	9.30
9.45	9.45	9.45
10.00	10.00	10.00
10.15	10.15	10.15
10.30	10.30	10.30
10.45	10.45	10.45
11.00	11.00	11.00
11.15	11.15	11.15
11.30	11.30	11.30
11.45	11.45	11.45
12.00	12.00	12.00
12.15	12.15	12.15
12.30	12.30	12.30
12.45	12.45	12.45
1.00	1.00	1.00
1.15	1.15	1.15
1.30	1.30	1.30
1.45	1.45	1.45
2.00	2.00	2.00
2.15	2.15	2.15
2.30	2.30	2.30
2.45	2.45	2.45
3.00	3.00	3.00
3.15	3.15	3.15
3.30	3.30	3.30
3.45	3.45	3.45
4.00	4.00	4.00
4.15	4.15	4.15
4.30	4.30	4.30
4.45	4.45	4.45
5.00	5.00	5.00
5.15	5.15	5.15
5.30	5.30	5.30

Month of_____ Week of_____to_____

THURSDAY /	FRIDAY /	SATURDAY /
8.00	8.00	
8.15	8.15	
8.30	8.30	
8.45	8.45	
9.00	9.00	
9.15	9.15	
9.30	9.30	
9.45	9.45	
10.00	10.00	
10.15	10.15	
10.30	10.30	
10.45	10.45	
11.00	11.00	
11.15	11.15	
11.30	11.30	
11.45	11.45	
12.00	12.00	
12.15	12.15	
12.30	12.30	
12.45	12.45	
1.00	1.00	SUNDAY /
1.15	1.15	
1.30	1.30	
1.45	1.45	
2.00	2.00	
2.15	2.15	
2.30	2.30	
2.45	2.45	
3.00	3.00	
3.15	3.15	
3.30	3.30	
3.45	3.45	
4.00	4.00	
4.15	4.15	
4.30	4.30	
4.45	4.45	
5.00	5.00	
5.15	5.15	
5.30	5.30	

Month of_____ Week of_____to_____

MONDAY /	TUESDAY /	WEDNESDAY /
8.00	8.00	8.00
8.15	8.15	8.15
8.30	8.30	8.30
8.45	8.45	8.45
9.00	9.00	9.00
9.15	9.15	9.15
9.30	9.30	9.30
9.45	9.45	9.45
10.00	10.00	10.00
10.15	10.15	10.15
10.30	10.30	10.30
10.45	10.45	10.45
11.00	11.00	11.00
11.15	11.15	11.15
11.30	11.30	11.30
11.45	11.45	11.45
12.00	12.00	12.00
12.15	12.15	12.15
12.30	12.30	12.30
12.45	12.45	12.45
1.00	1.00	1.00
1.15	1.15	1.15
1.30	1.30	1.30
1.45	1.45	1.45
2.00	2.00	2.00
2.15	2.15	2.15
2.30	2.30	2.30
2.45	2.45	2.45
3.00	3.00	3.00
3.15	3.15	3.15
3.30	3.30	3.30
3.45	3.45	3.45
4.00	4.00	4.00
4.15	4.15	4.15
4.30	4.30	4.30
4.45	4.45	4.45
5.00	5.00	5.00
5.15	5.15	5.15
5.30	5.30	5.30

Month of_____ Week of_____to_____

THURSDAY /	FRIDAY /	SATURDAY /
8.00	8.00	
8.15	8.15	
8.30	8.30	
8.45	8.45	
9.00	9.00	
9.15	9.15	
9.30	9.30	
9.45	9.45	
10.00	10.00	
10.15	10.15	
10.30	10.30	
10.45	10.45	
11.00	11.00	
11.15	11.15	
11.30	11.30	
11.45	11.45	
12.00	12.00	
12.15	12.15	
12.30	12.30	
12.45	12.45	
1.00	1.00	SUNDAY /
1.15	1.15	
1.30	1.30	
1.45	1.45	
2.00	2.00	
2.15	2.15	
2.30	2.30	
2.45	2.45	
3.00	3.00	
3.15	3.15	
3.30	3.30	
3.45	3.45	
4.00	4.00	
4.15	4.15	
4.30	4.30	
4.45	4.45	
5.00	5.00	
5.15	5.15	
5.30	5.30	

Month of_____ Week of_____to_____

MONDAY /	TUESDAY /	WEDNESDAY /
8.00	8.00	8.00
8.15	8.15	8.15
8.30	8.30	8.30
8.45	8.45	8.45
9.00	9.00	9.00
9.15	9.15	9.15
9.30	9.30	9.30
9.45	9.45	9.45
10.00	10.00	10.00
10.15	10.15	10.15
10.30	10.30	10.30
10.45	10.45	10.45
11.00	11.00	11.00
11.15	11.15	11.15
11.30	11.30	11.30
11.45	11.45	11.45
12.00	12.00	12.00
12.15	12.15	12.15
12.30	12.30	12.30
12.45	12.45	12.45
1.00	1.00	1.00
1.15	1.15	1.15
1.30	1.30	1.30
1.45	1.45	1.45
2.00	2.00	2.00
2.15	2.15	2.15
2.30	2.30	2.30
2.45	2.45	2.45
3.00	3.00	3.00
3.15	3.15	3.15
3.30	3.30	3.30
3.45	3.45	3.45
4.00	4.00	4.00
4.15	4.15	4.15
4.30	4.30	4.30
4.45	4.45	4.45
5.00	5.00	5.00
5.15	5.15	5.15
5.30	5.30	5.30

Month of_____ Week of_____to_____

THURSDAY /	FRIDAY /	SATURDAY /
8.00	8.00	
8.15	8.15	
8.30	8.30	
8.45	8.45	
9.00	9.00	
9.15	9.15	
9.30	9.30	
9.45	9.45	
10.00	10.00	
10.15	10.15	
10.30	10.30	
10.45	10.45	
11.00	11.00	
11.15	11.15	
11.30	11.30	
11.45	11.45	
12.00	12.00	
12.15	12.15	
12.30	12.30	
12.45	12.45	
1.00	1.00	SUNDAY /
1.15	1.15	
1.30	1.30	
1.45	1.45	
2.00	2.00	
2.15	2.15	
2.30	2.30	
2.45	2.45	
3.00	3.00	
3.15	3.15	
3.30	3.30	
3.45	3.45	
4.00	4.00	
4.15	4.15	
4.30	4.30	
4.45	4.45	
5.00	5.00	
5.15	5.15	
5.30	5.30	

Month of_____ Week of_____to_____

MONDAY /	TUESDAY /	WEDNESDAY /
8.00	8.00	8.00
8.15	8.15	8.15
8.30	8.30	8.30
8.45	8.45	8.45
9.00	9.00	9.00
9.15	9.15	9.15
9.30	9.30	9.30
9.45	9.45	9.45
10.00	10.00	10.00
10.15	10.15	10.15
10.30	10.30	10.30
10.45	10.45	10.45
11.00	11.00	11.00
11.15	11.15	11.15
11.30	11.30	11.30
11.45	11.45	11.45
12.00	12.00	12.00
12.15	12.15	12.15
12.30	12.30	12.30
12.45	12.45	12.45
1.00	1.00	1.00
1.15	1.15	1.15
1.30	1.30	1.30
1.45	1.45	1.45
2.00	2.00	2.00
2.15	2.15	2.15
2.30	2.30	2.30
2.45	2.45	2.45
3.00	3.00	3.00
3.15	3.15	3.15
3.30	3.30	3.30
3.45	3.45	3.45
4.00	4.00	4.00
4.15	4.15	4.15
4.30	4.30	4.30
4.45	4.45	4.45
5.00	5.00	5.00
5.15	5.15	5.15
5.30	5.30	5.30

Month of_____ Week of_____to_____

THURSDAY /	FRIDAY /	SATURDAY /
8.00	8.00	
8.15	8.15	
8.30	8.30	
8.45	8.45	
9.00	9.00	
9.15	9.15	
9.30	9.30	
9.45	9.45	
10.00	10.00	
10.15	10.15	
10.30	10.30	
10.45	10.45	
11.00	11.00	
11.15	11.15	
11.30	11.30	
11.45	11.45	
12.00	12.00	
12.15	12.15	
12.30	12.30	
12.45	12.45	
1.00	1.00	SUNDAY /
1.15	1.15	
1.30	1.30	
1.45	1.45	
2.00	2.00	
2.15	2.15	
2.30	2.30	
2.45	2.45	
3.00	3.00	
3.15	3.15	
3.30	3.30	
3.45	3.45	
4.00	4.00	
4.15	4.15	
4.30	4.30	
4.45	4.45	
5.00	5.00	
5.15	5.15	
5.30	5.30	